Keto Air Fryer Cookbook for Beginners

100 Keto Air Fryer Recipes for Body Healing and Easy Weight Loss (Keto Airfryer, Keto Air Fryer Recipes Cookbook, Air Fryer Ketogenic Recipes)

John Purcell

ISBN-13: 979- 8622050411

DEDICATION

To all who desire to live life to the fullest!

TABLE OF CONTENT

INTRODUCTION

It is no longer news that the ketogenic diet is a result-oriented diet. When implemented correctly, the corresponding outcome has always been rewarding. The ketogenic diet focuses on foods with heaps of healthy fat, very low carbs, and moderate amounts of protein. The ketogenic diet has many benefits, which includes: improvement of PCOS symptoms, reduction of seizures, protection of brain function, improvement of heart health, reduction of the susceptibility to some types of cancers, improvement of acne, supporting weight loss, increase in mental alertness and focus, increase in energy, less hunger, and more. The ketogenic diet has been tested, and proven over the years, and the results remain astounding.

Regrettably, the ketogenic diet like every other good diet can become pretty restraining on your preferred foods. Thankfully, the air fryer broadens your options with several keto air fryer recipes to prepare and choose from. The air fryer circulates hot air round your food and cooks it faster. Providing better tasting and healthy fried foods. The foods cooked are always tasty, golden brown, juicy and crispy. What's more? you can grill, fry, bake and roast your meals in the air fryer, opening you up to a whole new world of cooking for your keto meals. The Keto Air Fryer Cookbook for Beginners by John Purcell is an action-oriented, go-to cookbook filled with easy, delicious and healthy keto air fryer recipes that are high in healthy fats and very low in carbohydrates.

Each recipe in this book have been written with full nutritional information to help you keep track of the weight loss process without stress. Make the most of the information in this keto air fryer cookbook, and cook your way to optimal health and longevity.

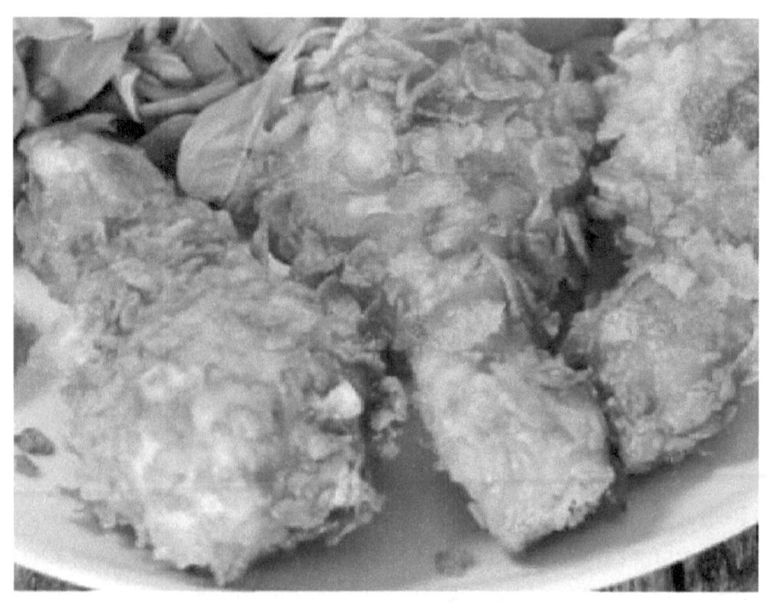

UNDERSTANDING THE AIR FRYER

The air fryer is a small convection oven that replicates the regular way of frying foods by passing hot air round the food instead of plunging the food in oil. These air fryer foods are usually tasteful, golden brown, juicy and crispy just like traditional frying. The foods that will be prepared in your air fryer, such as roasted veggies, baked seafood, crisped poultry, etc. will be better tasting and healthy. More often than not, the foods will be efficiently and quickly crisped.

The air fryer is nothing like a microwave oven, and it doesn't use radiation. The safety of air fryers without long-term damage from continuous use is a major health concern for most air fryer users. The heating element used in air fryers is comparable to those seen in a stovetop, toaster or any oven. Thus, the air fryer is a safe kitchen appliance that you can use without any fear of being exposed to any danger or side effects. The air fryer is a kitchen appliance that delivers when used according to manufacturer's instructions, and with the right recipes.

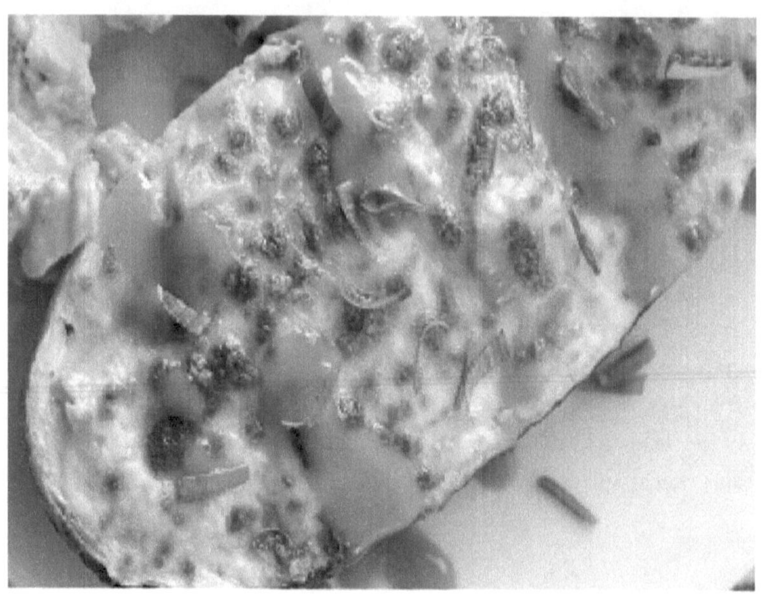

Benefits of Owning an Air Fryer

Given that the benefit of owning an air fryer is numerous, there are several reasons why you should consider having the air fryer:

Safety: The outer part of air fryer doesn't turn out to be hazardously hot, thus it is safe to touch and will not scald your hands. Similarly, unlike regular deep fryers, the air fryer does not hold large amounts of oil, therefore eliminating any chance of oil spills and burns.

Easy Cleaning: Seeing as the air fryer is enclosed, the air fryer enclosure stops spills and splatters that have a lot to do with pan frying and deep frying. What's more? The pans and wire baskets of a good number of air fryers are easy to clean and are dishwasher safe.

Clear-Cut and Ease of Use: Working the air fryer is as simple as tossing and coating your food in oil (if necessary), moving the food into the wire basket and allowing the air fryer to do the rest. Also, there are no fancy buttons/controls that requires schooling to operate. The digital display, knobs and controls for temperature and cook time are easy to understand and operate.

Saves Time: The air fryer cooks your food quicker than other regular methods of cooking. It pre-heats faster than convectional ovens, and comes to temperature in a matter of minutes.

Energy Efficiency: The air fryer is a kitchen appliance that is energy efficient. Cooking with it implies shorter cooking time, therefore less power is used.

Cooking Speed: The air fryer heats up and cooks quicker than regular ovens. Your foods will be crisped, juicy, golden brown and tasty in record time!

Healthy Cooking: For some reasons, such as health, most people have to keep away from deep-fried foods. The air fryer is a healthier-option since it uses 75% less oil than in pan frying or deep frying. The air fryer offers a healthy substitute without forfeiting flavor

Air Fryer Buying Tips

The following are things to look out for when considering which air fryer to buy:

Air Fryer Size: One of the factors that has to be put into consideration is the size of the air fryer that will suit your need. There are small and large air fryers, ranging from 2.2 qts. to 16 qts. models.

Air Fryer Features: The features and qualities of each air fryer differs. Research and buy an air fryer that has your desired features.

Guide to Using Air Fryer Oils

Since the air fryer is a healthy alternative to deep frying, most deep fryer recipes can be made in the air fryer with less oil. A good number of air fryer recipes call for approximately 1 tbsp of oil sprayed over the food before air frying. Some fatty foods, such as bacon, don't need to be sprayed with oil.

Nevertheless, leaner meats will need misting with oil to prevent sticking to the air fryer basket.

Oil misters or spray bottles are necessary equipment needed to coat food with the right amount of oil, just before it is cooked in the air fryer. Oils that can stand high temperatures before they burn are recommended. These oils have a high smoke point and will work well with your oil mister/spray bottles. Examples of such oils are:

Avocado Oil: Avocado oil adds a brilliant flavor to your food, with a high smoke point of 570°F.

Grapeseed oil: These oils can be used to dress, marinate, saute and cook your food. They are a great option when considering the type of oil to use while cooking air fryer recipes.

Refined Coconut Oil: This oil will add a distinct and delicious flavor to your food, and has a high smoke point of 450°F.

Light Olive Oil: The olive oil is also a great choice to use with your air fryer, and has a high smoke point of 468°F.

Peanut Oil: This nutty oil will give a yummy nutty flavor to your cooking, and it has a high smoke point of 450°F.

What Foods Can You Cook with the Air Fryer?

The air fryer can handle approximately 2-6 servings of food each time. The following foods can be cooked with the air fryer: tender, juicy steaks, fish and other seafood, bacon, keto hamburgers, turkey and chicken, keto donut holes, keto spring rolls, egg rolls, keto empanadas, one-serving pizzas, roasted veggies, grilled cheese keto sandwiches, baked zucchini chips, keto onion rings, keto tater tots and more.

The options of food that can be cooked in an air fryer is almost a never-ending one with boundless possibilities. As you become familiar with the air fryer, you will discover more recipes that can be made in your air fryer.

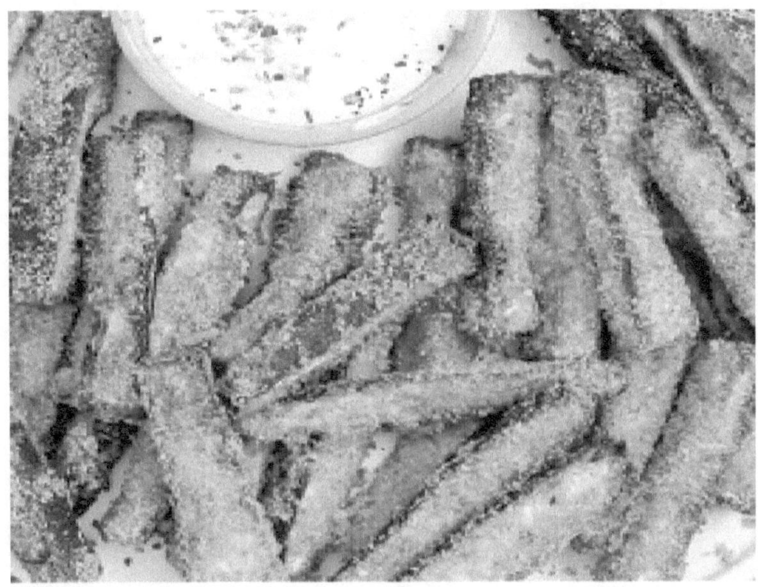

BREAKFAST

Air Fried Mozzarella Bread

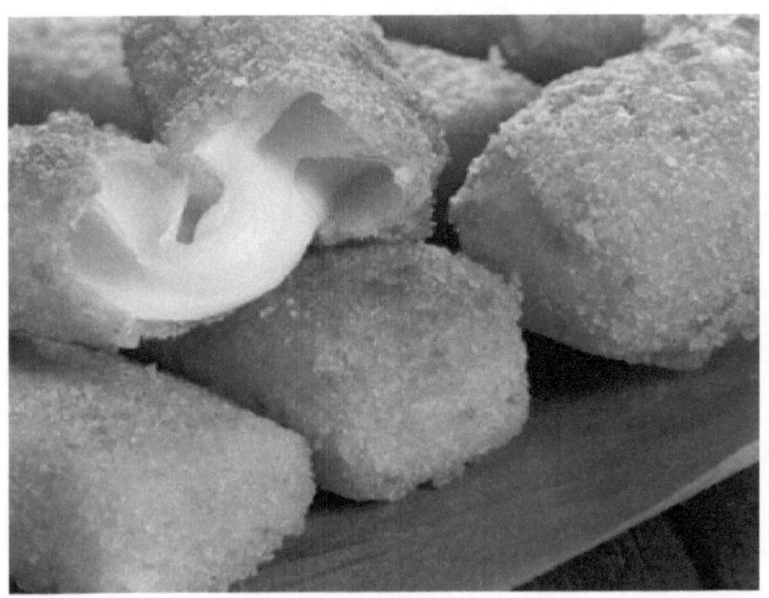

Preparation Time: 5 minutes

Cook Time: 10 minutes

Serves: 2 servings

Ingredients

1/4 cup Parmesan cheese, grated

1 cup mozzarella cheese, shredded

1/2 tsp garlic powder

1 egg, large

Method

1. Prepare a parchment paper lined air fryer basket. Add garlic powder, egg, parmesan cheese and mozzarella cheese into a bowl and mix well to combine. Mold mixture until a round-flat bread is formed. Place on the parchment paper lined basket.

2. Cook for 10 minutes at 350°F. Serve warm and dig in.

Nutritional Information/Serving

Calories 225 kcal, Protein 20.8g, Carbs 2.7g, Fat 14.3g

Hard-Boiled Eggs

Preparation Time: 2 minutes

Cook Time: 20 minutes

Serves: 6 servings

Ingredients

6 eggs, large

Method

1. Add the eggs into the wired basket of an air fryer and cook at 250°F for 19 minutes. Place cooked eggs under cold running water and peel off shell. Serve and enjoy.

Nutritional Information/Serving

Calories 62 kcal, Fat 4g, Protein 5g, Carbs 0g

Crispy Bacon

Preparation Time: 5 minutes

Cook Time: 10 minutes

Serves: 10 servings

Ingredients

10 bacon slices

Method

1. Add half of the bacon slices into the wired basket of an air fryer. Seal air fryer lid and cook until desired doneness is reached, for 10 minutes at 400°F. Use a tongue to flip bacon midway during cooking for even doneness.

2. Repeat process with the remaining bacon slices.

Nutritional Information/Serving

Calories 40 kcal, Protein 2.5g, Carbs 0g, Fat 3.5g

Morning Frittata

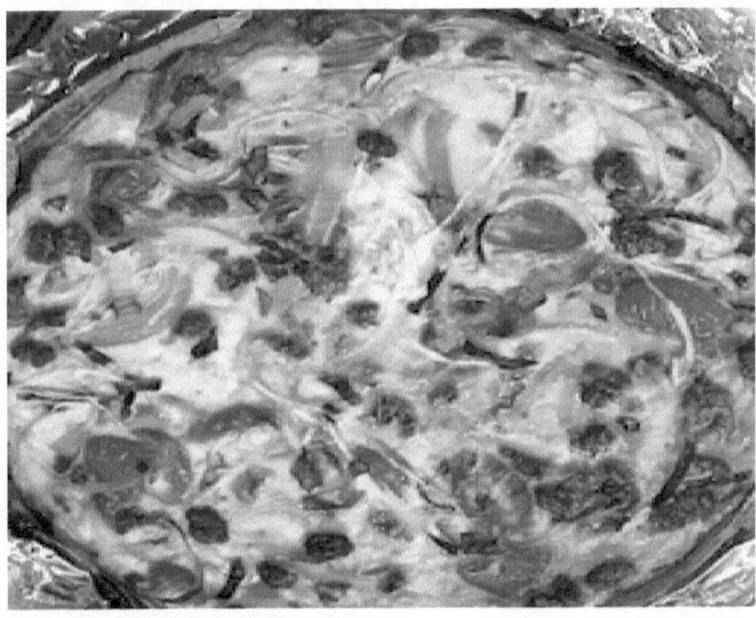

Preparation Time: 4 minutes

Cook Time: 16 minutes

Serves: 4 servings

Ingredients

3 tbsps heavy cream

4 eggs

4 (sliced) mushrooms

4 tbsps cheddar cheese, grated

4 tbsps kale, chopped

3 (halved) grape tomatoes

1 (sliced) green onion

2 tbsps fresh chopped cilantro

Salt

Method

1. Heat up air fryer to 350°F. Grease a parchment paper lined 7" baking pan and let sit. Add heavy cream and egg into a bowl and whisk until combined. Add every other ingredient into the cream mixture and stir until combined.

2. Pour mixture into the prepared baking pan. Move baking pan into the wire basket of an air fryer and cook until eggs are set, for 12-16 minutes. Check for doneness. Note: frittata is well cooked if an inserted toothpick in the middle of the frittata comes out clean.

Nutritional Information/Serving

Calories 147 kcal, Dietary Fiber 1g, Fat 11g, Protein 9g, Carbs 3g

Filled Peppers

Preparation Time: 5 minutes

Cook Time: 15 minutes

Serves: 2 servings

Ingredients

4 eggs

1 (halved lengthways; remove seeds) bell pepper

1 pinch salt and pepper

1 teaspoon avocado oil

Method

1. Coat pepper boats with avocado oil. Break 2 eggs into each bell pepper boat. Season filled pepper boats with pepper and salt. Transfer the filled pepper boats to the wire basket of an air fryer and cook for 13 minutes at 390°F

Nutritional Information/Serving

Calories 164 kcal, Protein 11g, Carbs 4g, Fat 10g

LUNCH

Air Fried Spicy Broccoli

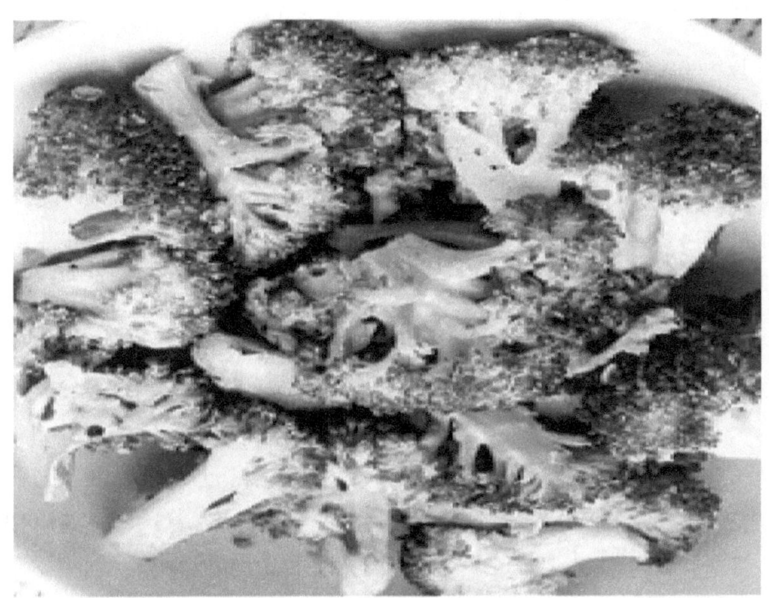

Preparation Time: 10 minutes

Cook Time: 20 minutes

Serves: 4 servings

Ingredients

1 1/2 tablespoons avocado oil

1 pound (cut into florets) broccoli

Salt

1 tablespoon minced garlic

2 teaspoons liquid stevia

2 tablespoons soy sauce, reduced sodium

1 teaspoon rice vinegar

2 teaspoons sriracha

Lemon juice

1/3 cup salted almonds, roasted

Method

1. Add garlic, avocado oil, broccoli and salt into a big bowl and toss until mixture is combined and the florets are wholly coated. Add mixture into the air fryer basket and spread evenly in one layer for even cooking.

2. Cook the broccoli mixture for about 15-20 minutes, until crispy and golden brown, at 400°F. Stir mixture midway while cooking. Note: Leave as much space as possible between the florets.

3. In the meantime, add rice vinegar, sriracha, soy sauce and stevia into a small oven-safe bowl, stir to combine and heat in a microwave until mixture melts together, for 10-15 seconds.

4. Move the air fried broccoli mixture into a serving bowl and top with the stevia-sauce. Toss mixture until coated and sprinkle with more salt as necessary. Top with lemon juice and roasted almonds and stir until combined.

Nutritional Information/Serving

Calories 233 kcal, Protein 8.1g, Carbs 12.5g, Fat 17.2g

Gouda Bacon Burger

Preparation Time: 10 minutes

Cook Time: 25 minutes

Serves: 2 servings

Ingredients

2 tbsps stevia

2 tbsps vanilla extract

¾ lb. (80% lean) ground beef

3 strips (halved) bacon

2 tbsps bbq sauce

1 tbsp onion, minced

Freshly ground black pepper, to taste

½ tsp salt

2 gouda cheese slices

Sauce

2 tbsps mayo

2 tbsps bbq sauce

Freshly ground black pepper, to taste

¼ tsp ground paprika

Serving

2 keto rolls/buns

Tomato

Lettuce

Method

1. Heat up air fryer to 390°F. Add little amount water into the drawer of the air fryer. Add stevia and vanilla extract not a bowl and combine. Add strips

of bacon into the wire basket of the air fryer and coat with the stevia-vanilla mixture.

2. Cook bacon for 4 minutes at 390°F. Turn, coat with extra stevia-vanilla mixture and cook until crisped, for 4 more minutes. In the meantime, add pepper, salt, BBQ sauce, onion and ground beef into a big bowl and combine.

3. Form ground beef mixture into 2 patties. Place patties into the wire basket of your air fryer and cook until desired doneness is reached, for 15-20 minutes at 370°F. Turn burgers midway while air frying.

4. Add black pepper, paprika, mayo and BBQ sauce into a bowl and combine for the sauce. Add a gouda cheese slice over each burger patty and cook until cheese is melted, for 1 more minute in the air fryer.

5. Spread sauce inside keto buns or rolls and top with burger, tomato lettuce and vanilla cooked bacon.

Nutritional Information/Serving

Calories 764 kcal, Protein 51.1g, Total Carbs 10.4g, Fat 52.2g

Crisped Pecorino Aubergines

Preparation Time: 15 minutes

Cook Time: 25 minutes

Serves: 4 servings

Ingredients

1/2 cup pork rind crumbs

1 (slice coarsely into 1/2" slices) eggplant, large

Salt, as necessary

3 tablespoons pecorino romano cheese, finely grated

3 tablespoons almond flour

1 teaspoon Italian seasoning

Avocado oil

1 tablespoon water + 1 egg

1/4 cup mozzarella cheese, grated

1 cup marinara sauce

2 tbsps cilantro

Method

1. Sprinkle eggplant slices with salt, rub in and let sit for about 15 minutes. In the meantime, add water and egg into a bowl and mix. Add in the almond flour and mix until a batter consistency is reached.

2. Add salt, Italian seasoning, pecorino Romano cheese and pork rinds into an average flat-bottomed bowl and stir well until combined. Dip eggplant slices into the batter until evenly covered. Immerse coated eggplant slices into the pork rind mixture until wholly coated.

3. Transfer eggplant slices into a platter and coat evenly with avocado oil. Heat up air fryer to 360°F. Add the breaded eggplant slices on the air fryer basket and cook for 8 minutes. Add mozzarella cheese and 1 tbsp marinara sauce over eggplant slices and cook until cheese is melted, for 1-2 more minutes.

4. Serve as desired and dig in.

Nutritional Information/Serving

Calories 227 kcal, Protein 11.9g, Total Carbs 8.2g, Fat 17

Delicious Air Fried Lasagna

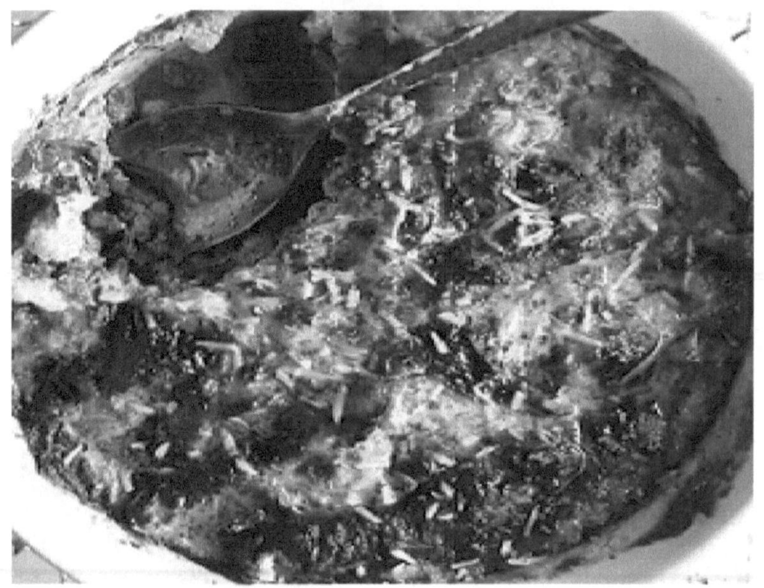

Preparation Time: 15 minutes

Cook Time: 30 minutes

Serves: 4 servings

Ingredients

1 (sliced into thin long slices) zucchini

1 cup marinara sauce

Sausage Layer

1 tsp garlic, minced

1 cup white onion, diced

1/2 lb. mild Italian sausage

Cheese Layer

1/2 cup mozzarella cheese, shredded

1/2 cup ricotta cheese

1 egg

1/2 cup (divided) parmesan, shredded

1/2 tsp dried Italian seasoning

1/2 tsp minced garlic

1/2 tsp black pepper

Method

1. Spray avocado oil into 7" springform pan. Lay zucchini slices into the prepared pan in intersecting layers. Top zucchini slices with 1/4 cup marinara sauce and spread until layer is covered evenly.

2. Add Italian sausage, garlic and onions into a big bowl and combine. Lay sausage over marinara layer and spread until layer is covered evenly. Top layer with the remaining marinara sauce and spread until layer is covered evenly.

3. Add 1/4 cup parmesan cheese, and the mozzarella cheese and ricotta into a clean bowl and combine. Top meat/marinara layer with cheese mixture and spread until layer is covered evenly.

4. Add the remaining parmesan cheese over cheese layer. Place a foil lid over springform pan and transfer into the fryer basket. Cook lasagna for 20 minutes at 350°. Get rid of the foil, cook until bubbly and the top becomes browned at 350°, for 8-10 minutes.

5. Let sit for 10 minutes until cooled before removing from the pan.

Nutritional Information/Serving

Calories 357 kcal, Protein 17g, Dietary Fiber 1g, Carbs 8g, Fat 27g

DESSERT

Air Fryer Cheesecake Bites

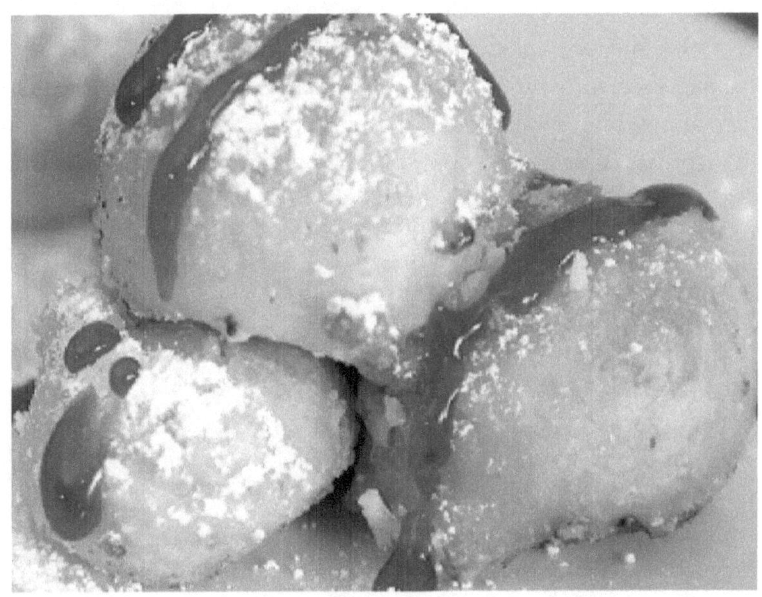

Preparation Time: 20 minutes

Cook Time: 2 minutes

Serves: 16 servings

Ingredients

1/2 cup erythritol

8 oz. cream cheese

1/2 tsp vanilla extract

4 tbsps (divided) heavy cream

2 tbsps erythritol

1/2 cup almond flour

Method

1. Set cream cheese aside to sit for 20 minutes until tender. Mix heavy cream, vanilla, 1/2 cup erythritol and softened cream cheese using a paddle attached-stand mixer until a smooth consistency is reached.

2. Scoop mixture onto a baking sheet lined with parchment paper. Transfer baking sheet into a freezer until solid, for 30 minutes. Add 2 tbsps erythritol and almond flour into a bowl and mix well. Immerse cheesecake bites into 2 tbsps heavy cream and coat with the erythritol-almond mixture.

3. Transfer cheesecake bites into the wire basket of an air fryer and cook for 2 minutes at 300°F.

Nutritional Information/Serving

Calories 80 kcal, Protein 2g, Carbs 2g, Fat 7g

Air Fryer Coconut Pie

Preparation Time: 10 minutes

Cook Time: 15 minutes

Serves: 8 servings

Ingredients

1 1/2 cups coconut milk

2 eggs

1 1/2 teaspoon vanilla extract

1/4 cup butter

1/2 cup monk fruit

1 cup coconut, shredded

1/2 cup coconut flour

Method

1. Prepare a 6" nonstick coated pie plate and let sit. Add every ingredient into a bowl and mix until combined. Fill the prepared pie plate with batter. Transfer pie plate into an air fryer and cook until an inserted toothpick comes out clean, for 10-12 minutes at 350°F.

2. Let sit to cool and garnish with keto sweetener powder and shredded coconut.

Nutritional Information/Serving

Calories 168 kcal, Protein 4.6g, Net Carbs 8.6g, Dietary Fiber 7.7g, Fat 10.7g

Molten Chocolate Cake

Preparation Time: 10 minutes

Cook Time: 10 minutes

Serves: 2 servings

Ingredients

2 tbsps cocoa powder

1 egg

2 tbsps erythritol, non-GMO

2 tbsps water

1 tbsp golden flax meal

1/8 tsp stevia

1/2 tsp baking powder, aluminum-free

1 tbsp melted coconut oil

1 pinch salt

1 dash of vanilla

Method

1. Add every ingredient into a ramekin or glass dish and whisk until combined. For 1 minute, heat up air fryer to 350°F. Place ramekin into the preheated air fryer and bake for 8-9 minutes. Cautiously take out ramekin or glass dish from the air fryer and let sit to cool.

2. Serve and enjoy.

Nutritional Information/Serving

Calories 126 kcal, Protein 4.9g, Total Carbs 2.3g, Fat 11.4g

BEEF

Filet Mignon Steak Skewers

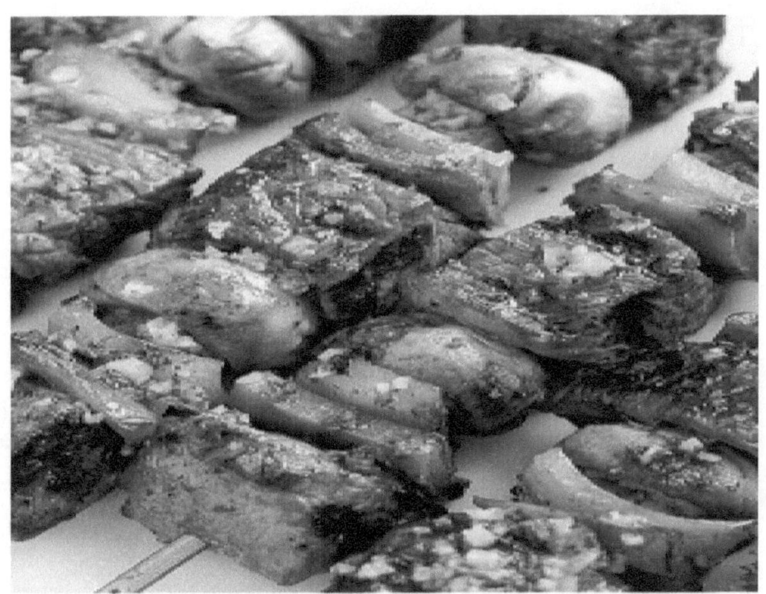

Preparation Time: 10 minutes

Cook Time: 12 minutes

Serves: 4 servings

Ingredients

¼ cup avocado oil

1 pound (cut into 1" chunks) filet mignon steak

1 tablespoon minced garlic

¼ cup soy sauce

½ teaspoon cumin, ground

1 teaspoon stevia

8 ounces (remove stems) baby bella mushrooms

¼ teaspoon black pepper

1 (chop into 1" pieces) green bell pepper

1 (chop into 1" pieces) red onion

Salt and pepper, as necessary

Method

1. Add black pepper, salt, cumin, garlic, stevia, soy sauce, avocado oil and steak into a big bowl, mix until well combined, and let sit for 30 minutes until marinated.

2. Alternatingly thread red onion, green pepper, mushrooms and the meat onto pre-soaked bamboo skewers. Heat up air fryer to 390°F. Add in the steak skewers to the basket of the preheated air fryer and cook for 5-6 minutes.

3. Flip skewers and cook for 5-6 more minutes.

Nutritional Information/Serving

Calories 320 kcal, Fat 18g, Protein 28g, Carbs 9g

Mushroom Steak Nuggets

Preparation Time: 10 minutes

Cook Time: 20 minutes

Serves: 4 servings

Ingredients

8 ounces (clean, wash and cut into halves) mushrooms

1 pound (cut into 1" cubes and pat dry) steaks

1 tsp Worcestershire sauce

2 tbsp melted butter

Salt and black pepper, as necessary

1/2 tsp garlic powder

Garnish with

Fresh minced cilantro

Method

1. Add mushrooms and cubed meats into a bowl and mix until combined. Add melted butter into the meat mixture until toss until coated. Sprinkle pepper, salt, garlic powder and Worcestershire sauce over mixture over mixture. For 4 minutes, heat up air fryer to 400°F.

2. Add the mushroom-meat mixture into the basket of the preheated air fryer in one layer. Cook for 10-18 minutes at 400°F. Flip and shake air fryer basket thrice while cooking. Check for doneness and cook for 2-5 more minutes, if necessary.

3. Serve warm, garnished with fresh minced cilantro.

Nutritional Information/Serving

Calories 198 kcal, Protein 23.9g, Carbs 3.5g, Fat 9.8g

Yummy Beef Satay with Roasted Pistachios

Preparation Time: 5 minutes

Cook Time: 8 minutes

Serves: 2 servings

Ingredients

2 tbsps avocado oil

1 lb. (cut into thin long strips) beef flank steak

1 tbsp soy sauce

1 tbsp fish sauce

1 tbsp garlic, minced

1 tbsp ginger, minced

1 tsp sriracha sauce

1 tbsp liquid stevia

1/2 cup (divided) parsley, chopped

1 tsp coriander, ground

1/4 cup (roasted) pistachios, chopped

Method

1. Add beef into a big bowl. Add 1/4 cup parsley, coriander, sriracha, stevia, garlic, ginger, soy sauce, fish sauce and avocado oil into the big bowl and mix until combined.

2. Refrigerate beef mixture for 30 minutes until marinated. Transfer beef into the wire basket of an air fryer in one single layer. Get rid of excess marinade. Cook beef for 8 minutes at 360°F. Turn beef midway while cooking. Transfer into a platter and top with roasted pistachios and 1/4 cup chopped parsley.

3. Serve and dig in.

Nutritional Information/Serving

Calories 582 kcal, Fat 34g, Protein 56g, Carbs 12g

Carne Asada with Grapefruit

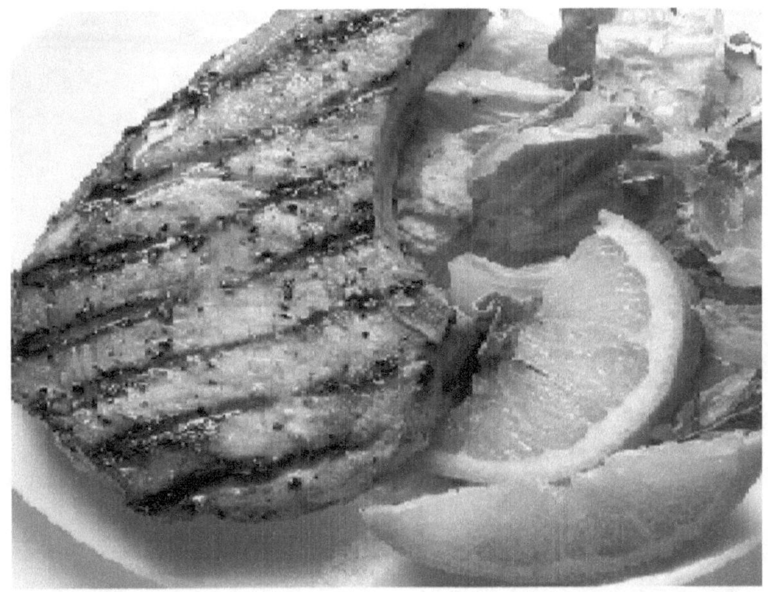

Preparation Time: 10 minutes

Cook Time: 8 minutes

Serves: 4 servings

Ingredients

1 medium (peeled and seeded) grapefruit

2 medium (juiced) limes

1 (diced) jalapeño pepper

1 cup parsley

2 tbsps white vinegar

2 tbsps avocado oil

1 tsps stevia

2 tsps ancho chile powder

1 tsp cumin seeds

1 tsp salt

1 1/2 lbs. skirt steak

1 tsp coriander seeds

Method

1. Add every ingredient into a high-speed electric blender, excluding the skirt steak. Blend mixture until a smooth consistency is reached. Slice steak into 4 portions and move into a Ziploc bag.

2. Add the blended marinade into the Ziploc bag, shake and refrigerate for 1-8 hours until marinated. Heat up air fryer to 400°F. Work in batches, transfer the marinated steaks into the wire basket of an air fryer in a single layer.

3. Cook until steak reaches an internal temperature of 145°F, for 8 minutes. Let sit to cool before serving.

Nutritional Information/Serving

Calories 330 kcal, Fat 19g, Protein 37g, Carbs 1g

Scrumptious Beef-loaf Sliders

Preparation Time: 10 minutes

Cook Time: 10 minutes

Serves: 8 servings

Ingredients

2 (beaten) eggs

1 pound ground beef

1 minced garlic clove

¼ cup (chopped finely) onion

¼ cup coconut flour

½ cup (extra-fine) almond flour, blanched

½ teaspoon sea salt

¼ cup ketchup

1 tablespoon Worcestershire Sauce

½ teaspoon black pepper

½ teaspoon dried dill

1 teaspoon Italian seasoning

Method

1. Add every ingredient into a big bowl and mix until well combined. Form 1" thick and 2" wide patties from the mixture. Transfer patties into a refrigerator for 10 minutes to firm up. Heat up air fryer to 360°F. Work in batches, add in patties into the air fryer basket.

2. Seal the lid and air fry for 10 minutes. Midway during cooking, check the patties. Repeat process with the remaining patties. Serve with roasted vegetables or keto salad.

Nutritional Information/Serving

Calories 228 kcal, Protein 13g, Carbs 4g, Fat 5g

Delicious Beef Steak Bites

Preparation Time: 15 minutes

Cook Time: 20 minutes

Serves: 4 servings

Ingredients

1 egg, large

1 lb. (cut into chunks) beef steak

Avocado oil

Ranch Dip

1/4 cup sour cream

1/4 cup mayo

1/2 tsp ranch dressing

1 tsp chipotle paste

1/4 (juiced) lemon, medium

Breading

1/2 cup pork rind

1/2 cup parmesan cheese, grated

1/2 tsp seasoned salt

Method

1. Add every ranch dip ingredient into a bowl and mix until well combined. Place mixture into a refrigerator for 30 minutes-7 days. Add seasoned salt, parmesan cheese and pork rind into a bowl, combine and let sit.

2. Heat up air fryer to 400°F. Add 1 egg into a bowl and beat well. Immerse steak pieces into the egg wash and dip into the pork rind bowl until wholly covered. Transfer breaded steak chunks onto a baking pan lined with parchment paper.

3. Transfer pan with steak into a freezer for 30 minutes. Coat the wired basket of an air fryer with avocado oil and add the chilled chunks of steaks in a single layer. Seal air fryer lead and cook for 5 minutes. Flip steals and cook for 2-3 more minutes.

4. Season with extra salt, let sit to cool and serve with ranch dip.

Nutritional Information/Serving

Calories 350 kcal, Fat 20g, Protein 40g, Carbs 1g

Beef Bulgogi with Scallion-Mayo Sauce

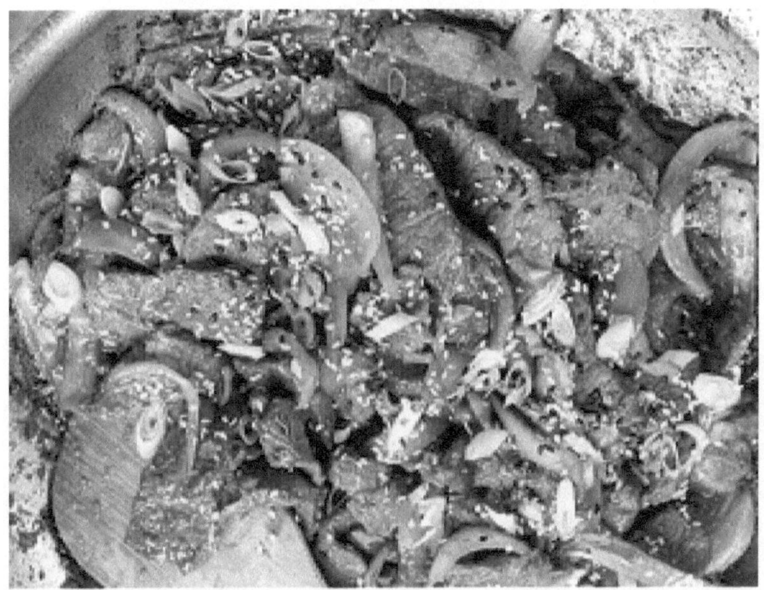

Preparation Time: 15 minutes

Cook Time: 10 minutes

Serves: 4 servings

Ingredients (beef)

2 tbsp gochujang

1 lb. ground beef, lean

2 tsp garlic, minced

1 tbsp dark soy sauce

2 tsp stevia

2 tsp ginger, minced

1/4 cup green onions

1 tbsp sesame Oil

1/2 teaspoon salt

Scallion-Mayo Sauce

1 tbsp gochujang

1/4 cup mayonnaise

2 tsp sesame seeds

1 tbsp sesame oil

1/4 cup (chopped) scallions

Method

1. Add salt, chopped onions, sesame oil, stevia, ginger, garlic, soy sauce, gochujang and ground beef into a big bowl, mix until combined and refrigerate for 1-8 hours.

2. Form mixture into 4 round patties and make an indentation in the center of each patty. Transfer patties into the wire basket of an air fryer in one layer, and cook for 10 minutes at 360°F.

3. In the meantime, add every mayo sauce ingredient into a bowl and mix until well combined. Serve beef bulgogi with scallion-mayo sauce over keto burgers or as is.

Nutritional Information/Serving

Calories 392 kcal, Fat 29g, Protein 24g, Cards 7g

Ribeye Steak with Herb Butter

Preparation Time: 20 minutes

Cook Time: 15 minutes

Serves: 2 servings

Ingredients

Salt and freshly cracked black pepper

2 (8 ounces) Ribeye steak, at room temperature

Avocado oil

Herbed Butter

2 tablespoons fresh chopped cilantro

1 stick (softened) butter, unsalted

1 teaspoon Worcestershire Sauce

2 teaspoons minced garlic

1/2 teaspoon salt

Method

1. Add every ingredient for the herb butter into a bowl and mix until well combined. Add into a parchment sheet and roll until a log is formed. Place in a refrigerator to chill before serving.

2. Coat steak with avocado oil until evenly covered on both sides and sprinkle with freshly cracked black pepper and salt. Coat the wired basket of an air fryer and heat up to 400°F. Add steak into the preheated air fryer basket.

3. Seal the lid and cook for 6 minutes, flip and cook for 6 more minutes, for medium cooked steak.

Nutritional Information/Serving

Calories 579 kcal, Protein 29.5g, Total Carbs 2.5g, Fat 49.5g

Spicy Chuck Steak with Cocoa

Preparation Time: 20 minutes

Cook Time: 10 minutes

Serves: 2 servings

Ingredients

1 1/2 teaspoons sea salt, coarse

1 pound chuck steak

1/2 teaspoon coffee, ground

1 teaspoon brown sugar

1/4 teaspoon chili powder

1/2 teaspoon black pepper

1/4 teaspoon onion powder

1/4 teaspoon garlic powder

1/4 teaspoon chipotle powder

1/4 teaspoon paprika

1/8 teaspoon cocoa powder

1/8 teaspoon coriander

Method

1. Add every spice into a small bowl, including cocoa and coffee and whisk until broken up and combined. Pour a liberal amount of the spice mixture

onto a platter. Coat and rub steak into the spice mixture until evenly covered.

2. Turn steak over and coat well on the other side. Coat the wired basket of an air fryer with avocado oil. For 3 minutes, heat up air fryer to 390°F. Place steak in the prepared air fryer basket, seal and cook for 9 minutes. Note: don't open basket or flip throughout the cooking.

3. Remove the cooked steak, let sit for 5 minutes, slice and serve.

Nutritional Information/Serving

Calories 495 kcal, Fay 32g, Protein 46g, Carbs 5g

PORK

Baby Back Ribs

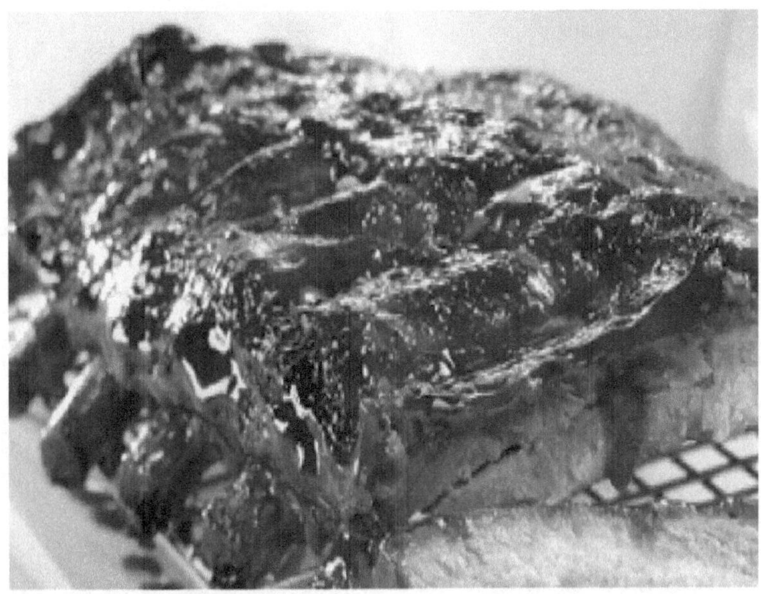

Preparation Time: 15 minutes

Cook Time: 35 minutes

Serves: 4 servings

Ingredients

1 tbsp avocado oil

1 rack (get rid of membrane from the back; pat dry and slice into 4 chunks) baby back ribs

1 tbsp stevia powder

1 tbsp liquid smoke

1/2 tsp black pepper, ground

1/2 tsp salt

1/2 tsp onion powder

1/2 tsp garlic powder

1 cup BBQ sauce

1/2 tsp chili powder

Method

1. Add liquid smoke and avocado oil into a small bowl and combine. Coat ribs evenly with the liquid smoke mixture. Add chili powder, onion powder, garlic powder, pepper, salt and stevia powder into a bowl and combine.

2. Sprinkle seasoning mixture over ribs until wholly coated on every side. Let ribs sit until flavors are infused, for 30 minutes. Heat up air fryer to 375°F. Place the seasoned ribs in one layer on the wire basket of the air fryer.

3. Cook ribs for 15 minutes. Turn ribs and cook for 10 more minutes. Take out ribs from the air fryer and coat bone-side of baby back ribs with 1/2 cup BBQ sauce. Return ribs into the air fryer basket, cook for 5 minutes before flipping.

4. Coat the turned rib side (meat side) with the reserved 1/2 cup BBQ sauce and cook until charred as desired, for 5 more minutes.

Nutritional Information/Serving

Calories 445 kcal, Protein 18.2g, Carbs 26.8g, Fat 29g

Garlic Pork Chops with Cheese

Preparation Time: 10 minutes

Cook Time: 15 minutes

Serves: 6 servings

Ingredients

1 1/2 teaspoons garlic powder

1/2 cup parmesan cheese, grated

1 teaspoon sage, dried

1 tablespoon cilantro, dried

3/4 teaspoon salt

1 teaspoon paprika

1/2 teaspoon onion powder

1/2 teaspoon pepper

1/8 teaspoon basil

1/4 teaspoon chili powder

4 pork chops

1 tablespoon avocado oil

Method

1. Heat up air fryer to 380°F. Coat the basket of the air fryer with avocado oil. Add spices and parmesan cheese into a flat-bottomed bowl and whisk until well combined.

2. Add avocado oil into a big skillet over med-heat. Sprinkle spice mixture over pork until wholly coated. Cook until pork is seared on both sides. Transfer the seared pork into the preheated air fryer and cook until well cooked, for about 10-14 minutes at 380°F. Flip once during cooking.

Nutritional Information/Serving

Calories 423 kcal, Protein 59.8g, Carbs 4g, Fat 17.2g

Moist Pork Chops

Preparation Time: 2 minutes

Cook Time: 15 minutes

Serves: 4 servings

Ingredients

Salt and pepper, as necessary

4 (boneless; thick) pork chops

Method

1. Sprinkle pepper and salt over pork chops until liberally seasoned. Transfer pork chops into the wire basket of an air fryer in one layer. Cook for until pork chops are well cooked, for 10-15 minutes. Turn pork chops midway during cooking.

Nutritional Information/Serving

Calories 328 kcal, Protein 40g, Carbs 0g, Fat 17g

Pork Thit Nuong

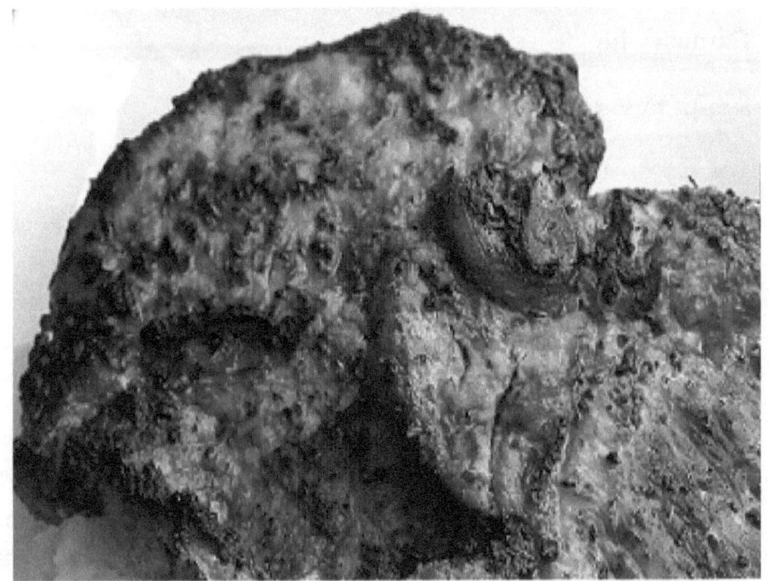

Preparation Time: 20 minutes

Cook Time: 10 minutes

Serves: 4 servings

Ingredients (marinade)

2 tbsps avocado oil

1/4 cup onions, minced

2 tsps dark soy sauce

1 tbsp splenda

1 tbsp fish sauce

1 tbsp garlic, minced

1/2 tsp pepper

1 tbsp (store-bought) minced lemongrass paste

1 lb. (sliced thin into small bite-sized pieces) pork shoulder

Garnish with

2 tbsps fresh chopped parsley

1/4 cup roasted peanuts, crumbled

Method

1. Add pepper, lemongrass paste, fish sauce, garlic, avocado oil, soy sauce, splenda and onions into a bowl and whisk to combine. Add pork pieces into the marinade, toss until coated and let sit for 30 minutes or more until marinated.

2. Place marinated pork into the fryer basket in one layer. Cook pork for 5 minutes at 400°. Flip pork and cook for 5 minutes until desired doneness is reached. Serve pork, garnished with fresh chopped parsley and crumbled peanuts.

Nutritional Information/Serving

Calories 231 kcal, Protein 16g, Dietary Fiber 1g, Carbs 4g, Fat 16g

Thick-Cut Bacon with Cabbage

Preparation Time: 10 minutes

Cook Time: 25 minutes

Serves: 6 servings

Ingredients

6 thick-cut bacon strips

1 (get rid of the outer layer before cutting cabbage into wedges) green cabbage head, small

1 teaspoon garlic powder

1 teaspoon onion powder

1/4 teaspoon chili flakes

1/2 teaspoon fennel seeds

Salt and pepper, as necessary

3 tablespoons avocado oil

Method

1. Liberally coat the wire basket of an air fryer with avocado oil. Add slices of bacon into the air fryer basket and cook for 10 minutes at 360°F. Cut cooked bacon slices into small pieces and let sit.

2. Add pepper, salt, chili flakes, fennel seeds, onion powder and garlic powder into a small bowl and mix until combined. Dribble avocado oil over cabbage and season with the garlic powder mixture until evenly covered.

3. Liberally grease the wire basket of an air fryer basket with avocado oil. Add in the seasoned cabbage wedges into the prepared air fryer basket and cook for 8 minutes at 400°F. Flip cabbage wedges, coat with extra avocado oil and cook for 6 more minutes.

4. Remove and let sit to cool. Serve, topped with chopped bacon.

Nutritional Information/Serving

Calories 123 kcal, Protein 4g, Carbs 2g, Fat 11g

Juicy Pork Chops

Preparation Time: 5 minutes

Cook Time: 15 minutes

Serves: 3 servings

Ingredients

2 tsps avocado oil

3 (6 oz.) {rinse and pat dry} pork chops

Black pepper, as necessary

Salt, as necessary

1 tsp smoked paprika, or to taste

1 tsp garlic powder, or to taste

Method

1. Coat the pork chops lightly with avocado oil. Sprinkle smoked paprika, garlic powder, pepper and salt over pork chops to season. Transfer pork chops into the wire basket of an air fryer, and cook for 5-7 minutes at 380°F.

2. Turn the pork chop and cook until well cooked, for 5-7 more minutes. Let sit to cool slightly before serving.

Nutritional Information/Serving

Calories 227 kcal, Protein 34.8g, Total Carbs 2.7g, Fat 9.8g

Air Fryer Pork Belly

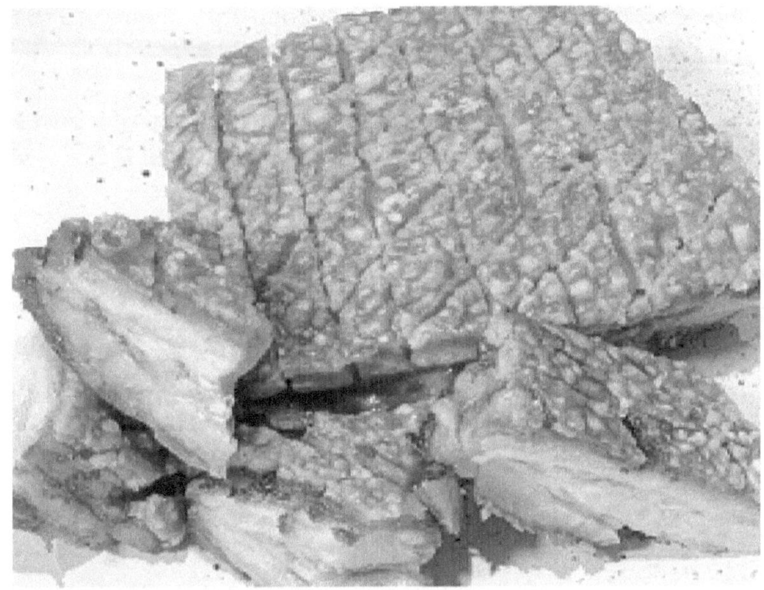

Preparation Time: 10 minutes

Cook Time: 30 minutes

Serves: 4 servings

Ingredients

3 cups water

1 lb. (cut into 3 chunks) pork belly

1 tsp black pepper, ground

1 tsp salt

2 bay leaves

2 tbsps soy sauce

6 garlic cloves

Method

1. Add every ingredient into a saucepan, place lid over pan and cook until a knife pierces the skin-side easily, for an hour. Take out meat, let sit for 10 minutes to dry and drain.

2. Slice each chunk of pork belly into 2 long slices. Transfer pork slices into the wire basket of an air fryer. Cook until pork belly fat is crispy, for 15 minutes at 400°F.

3. Serve and enjoy.

Nutritional Information/Serving

Calories 594 kcal, Fat 21g, Fat 60g, Protein 11g

POULTRY

Mushroom Chicken Patties

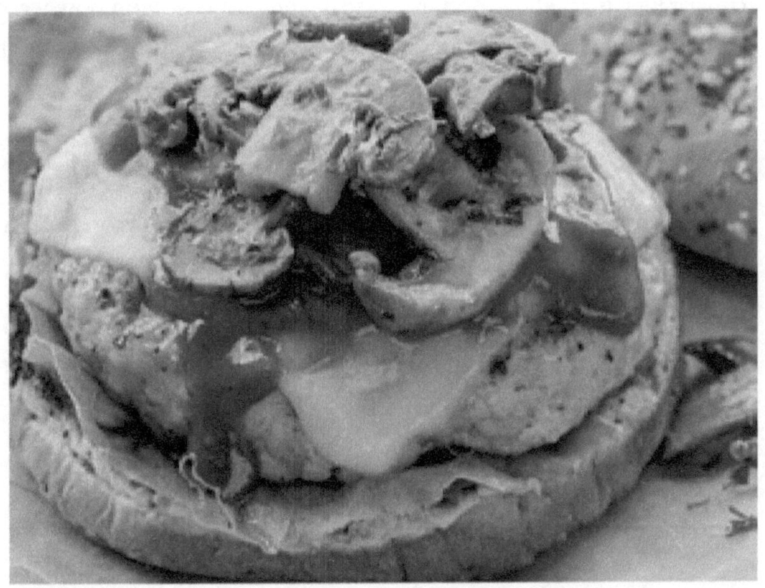

Preparation Time: 10 minutes

Cook Time: 10 minutes

Serves: 5 servings

Ingredients

1 tbsp seasoning sauce

6 medium (wash and shake excess liquid off) fresh mushrooms (30g ea)

1 tsp onion powder

1 tsp garlic powder

1/2 tsp black pepper, ground

1/2 tsp salt

500g chicken, ground extra lean.

Method

1. Add the washed mushrooms into a food processor and puree until a fine consistency is reached. Add in the seasoning sauce, onion powder, garlic powder, ground black pepper and salt into the food processor and process for a minute.

2. Pour the food processor mixture into a big bowl, and add in the ground chicken. Use clean hands to mix until well combined. Split mixture into 5 portions and shape into 5 even patties. Make an indentation in the middle of each patty.

3. Coat avocado oil on each side of each patty. Transfer patties into the wire basket of an air fryer in one layer. Cook until an internal temperature of 165°F is reached, for 10 minutes at 360°F.

4. Serve at once and dig in.

Nutritional Information/Serving

Calories 130 kcal, Protein 19.2g, Total Carbs 0.7g, Fat 9g

Air Fryer Chicken Strips

Preparation Time: 10 minutes

Cook Time: 15 minutes

Serves: 6 servings

Ingredients

4 tablespoons avocado oil

1 (whisked) egg

100g almond flour

850g (cut into strips) chicken breast

1/2 teaspoon garlic powder

1/2 teaspoon salt

1 teaspoon onion flakes

Method

1. Add avocado oil and egg into a bowl and whisk until combined. Add onion, garlic, salt and almond flour into a bowl and mix until combined. Immerse chicken strips into the avocado oil mixture until wholly coated.

2. Coat the wire basket of an air fryer with avocado oil. Add in the chicken strips and cook for 10 minutes at 350°F. Serve as desired.

Nutritional Information/Serving

Calories 445 kcal, Protein 48.8g, Carbs 4.5g, Fat 25.5g

Delicious Tandoori Turkey

Preparation Time: 20 minutes

Cook Time: 15 minutes

Serves: 4 servings

Ingredients

1/4 cup Greek yogurt

1 lb. (cut each in half) turkey tenders

1 tbsp garlic, minced

1 tbsp ginger, minced

1 tsp salt

¼ cup fresh chopped parsley

1 tsp turmeric

1/2 tsp cayenne pepper

1 tsp sweet smoked paprika

1 tsp garam masala

Garnish with

2 tbsp fresh chopped parsley

2 tsps lime juice

1 tbsp avocado oil

Method

1. Add every ingredient into a glass dish, excluding the garnish. Let mixture sit until marinated. For 5 minutes, heat up air fryer to 350°. Carefully arrange tandoori turkey into fryer basket in one layer.

2. Brush turkey with avocado oil on a side. Cook tandoori turkey for 10 minutes at 350°. Flip turkey, baste with extra avocado oil and cook until desired doneness is reached, for 5 more minutes.

3. Add parsley and lime juice into a bowl and combine. Move tandoori turkey to a platter and garnish with parsley mixture.

Nutritional Information/Serving

Calories 178 kcal, Protein 25g, Carbs 2g, Fat 6g

Crunchy Turkey with Mayonnaise

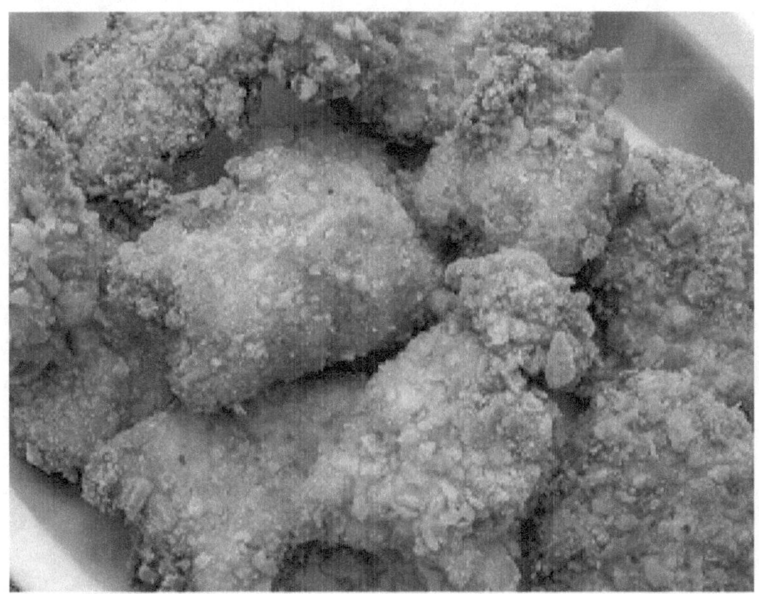

Preparation Time: 15 minutes

Cook Time: 10 minutes

Serves: 6 servings

Ingredients

4 ounces pork rinds, crushed

6 (pat dry) turkey thighs, boneless

2 teaspoons salt

2 teaspoons thyme, ground

1 teaspoon garlic powder

1 ½ teaspoons paprika

¼ teaspoon black pepper

¼ teaspoon cayenne pepper, ground

¼ cup mayonnaise

1 egg

1 tablespoon mustard

2 tablespoons hot sauce

Method

1. Heat up air fryer to 390°F. Add every dry ingredient into a small bowl and whisk until combined. Pour 1/2 of the dry mixture into a flat-bottomed bowl. Add mustard, hot sauce, mayonnaise and egg into a second bowl and mix until combined.

2. Immerse one turkey piece into the mayo-egg mixture until covered and transfer into the dry mixture until wholly and evenly coated. Move the breaded turkey pieces into the wire basket of the air fryer.

3. Repeat process until every turkey piece is wholly coated. Arrange in the air fryer basket in a single layer. Cook until an internal temperature of 165°F is reached, for 10 minutes.

4. Let turkey pieces sit to cool before you slice.

Nutritional Information/Serving

Calories 372 kcal, Protein 41.2g, Carbs 0.9g, Fat 23g

Yummy Chicken Roast

Preparation Time: 10 minutes

Cook Time: 50 minutes

Serves: 6 servings

Ingredients

1 pinch garlic salt

Ground black pepper

2 tbsps butter

1/3 cup salt

1/3 cup stevia powder

1 (3 lbs.) chicken breast, thawed

2 cups water

Method

1. Add 2 cups water into a saucepan over med-heat and bring to boiling. Add in pepper, Stevie powder and 1/3 cup salt and stir until combined. Take pan off heat and let sit for 30 minutes until wholly cool.

2. Add chicken into the pan with brine until wholly covered, place lid over bowl and refrigerate for 8 hours. Heat up air fryer to 390°F. Take chicken out of the brine and get rid of brine. Pat dry the chicken and smear with butter.

3. Sprinkle pepper and garlic salt over coated chicken. Place seasoned chicken in the wire basket of the preheated air fryer and cook for 15 minutes. Flip and sprinkle with garlic salt and pepper. Adjust air fryer temp to 360°F.

4. Cook chicken for 15 more minutes, flip and cook for 5 more minutes. Adjust air fryer temperature to 390°F, flip chicken again and cook for 15

more minutes, until no pink remains in the middle. Let chicken sit for 5 minutes. Slice chicken and serve as desired.

Nutritional Information/Serving

Calories 314 kcal, Protein 48g, Carbs 4g, Fat 9.8g

Turkey Breast Dinner

Preparation Time: 5 minutes

Cook Time: 15 minutes

Serves: 1 serving

Ingredients

1 teaspoon poultry seasoning

1 (7 ounces) {pat dry} turkey breast, skinless

Avocado oil

Method

1. Heat up air fryer to 390°F. Dribble avocado oil over turkey breast and sprinkle with poultry seasoning. Coat the wire basket of an air fryer with avocado oil until wholly covered. Add the turkey breast into the prepared air fryer and cook until an internal temperature of 165°F is reached, for 12-15 minutes.

2. Let cooked turkey breast sit to cool for 5 minutes. Serve and dig in.

Nutritional Information/Serving

Calories 262 kcal, Fat 6g, Protein 48g, Carbs 1g

Herbed Whole Turkey

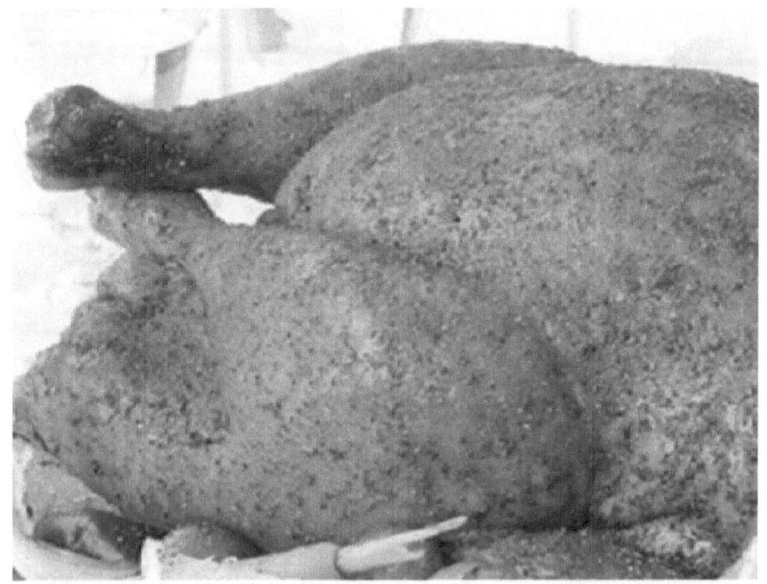

Preparation Time: 5 minutes

Cook Time: 60 minutes

Serves: 6 servings

Ingredients

2 tbsps avocado oil

1 (5 lbs.) {remove giblets} whole turkey

1 tsp black pepper, freshly ground

1 tbsp salt

1 tsp paprika

1 tsp garlic powder

1/2 tsp parsley, dried

1/2 tsp cilantro, dried

1/2 tsp sage, dried

Method

1. Add avocado oil, herb and seasoning into a bowl and mix until a pasty consistency is reached. Coat whole turkey with the paste mixture until evenly covered. Cover the wire basket of an air fryer with avocado oil.

2. Transfer the seasoned whole turkey into the prepared air fryer, with the breast side down. Air fryer for 50 minutes at 360°F. Turn turkey and cook until an internal temperature of 165°F is reached, for 10 more minutes.

3. Carve and slice turkey before serving.

Nutritional Information/Serving

Calories 444 kcal, Protein 60.2g, Total Carbs 21g, Fat 11.2g

Spicy Caribbean Turkey

Preparation Time: 10 minutes

Cook Time: 10 minutes

Serves: 8 servings

Ingredients

Salt and coarse ground black pepper, to taste

3 pounds (pat dried) Turkey thigh, skinless, boneless

1 tablespoon cinnamon, ground

1 tablespoon ground coriander seed

1 1/2 teaspoons ginger, ground

1 tablespoon cayenne pepper

3 tablespoons melted coconut oil

1 1/2 teaspoons nutmeg, ground

Method

1. Cover turkey on a big baking sheet with paper towels until remaining moisture is soaked up. Season turkey with pepper and salt until wholly covered. Let sit at room temperature for 30 minutes.

2. Add nutmeg, ginger, cayenne, cinnamon and coriander into a small bowl and mix until combined. Sprinkle nutmeg mixture over turkey until wholly coated and brush evenly with melted coconut oil.

3. Work in batches, add 4 (3-4 ounces ea) turkey pieces into the wire basket of an air fryer, and cook for 10 minutes at 390°F. Transfer into a heat-proof bowl and cover with aluminum foil. Let sit in an oven to keep warm.

4. Repeat process with the remaining turkey until wholly cooked. Serve turkey warm as desired.

Nutritional Information/Serving

Calories 202 kcal, Protein 24.9g, Carbs 1.7g, Fat 13.4g

Hot and Crisped Turkey Drumettes

Preparation Time: 10 minutes

Cook Time: 25 minutes

Serves: 6 servings

Ingredients

2 tsps soy sauce, low-sodium

16 turkey drumettes

1 teaspoon garlic powder

Italian seasoning, to taste

Avocado oil

Pepper, as necessary

1/4 cup buffalo wing sauce

Method

1. Evenly dribble soy sauce over turkey drumettes until coated. Sprinkle pepper, garlic powder and Italian seasoning over turkey as necessary. Move turkey meat into the wire basket of an air fryer and coat with avocado oil until wholly covered.

2. Cook at 400°F for 5 minutes. Take out the basket and shake for even cooking. Place back the wired basket into the air fryer and cook for 5 more minutes. Coat turkey with Buffalo sauce and cook until no pink remains and turkey is crisped as desired, for 7-12 more minutes.

3. Let sit to cool. Serve and enjoy.

Nutritional Information/Serving

Calories 208 kcal, Fat 16g, Protein 15g, Carbs 1g

Turkey Meatballs

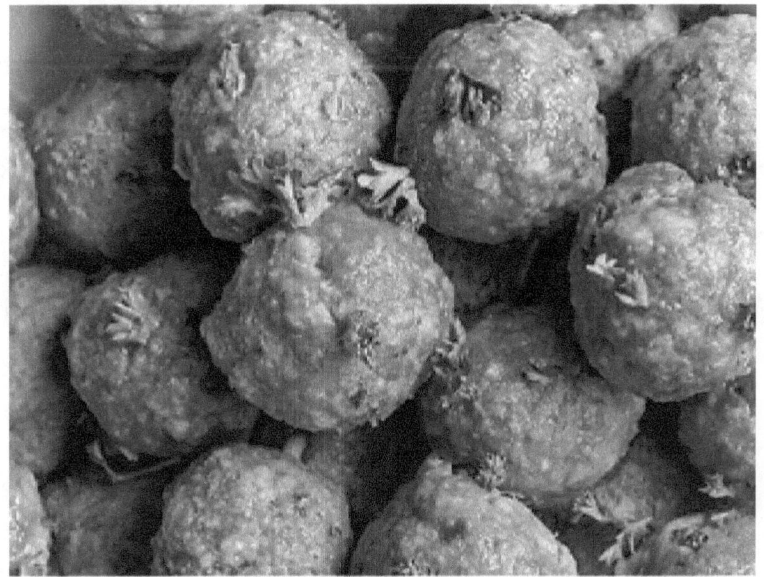

Preparation Time: 10 minutes

Cook Time: 15 minutes

Serves: 4 servings

Ingredients

2 (chop finely) green onions

1 lb. ground turkey

1 tbsp hoisin sauce

1/2 cup fresh chopped parsley

1 tsp sriracha sauce

1 tbsp soy sauce

1/4 cup shredded coconut, unsweetened

1 tsp sesame oil

Ground black pepper, as necessary

Salt, as necessary

Method

1. Add every ingredient into a bowl and mix until well combined. Scoop balls of the ground turkey mixture onto a parchment paper lined plate. Working in batches, transfer meatballs into the wire basket of an air fryer.

2. Seal the lid and cook at 350°F until an internal temperature of 165°F is reached, for 5 minutes. Flip and cook for 5 more minutes.

3. Adjust air fryer temperature to 400°F and cook for 2-3 more minutes, until meatballs are brown.

Nutritional Information/Serving

Calories 223 kcal, Fat 14g, Protein 20g, Carbs 3g

Chicken Drumsticks

Preparation Time: 5 minutes

Cook Time: 25 minutes

Serves: 2 servings

Ingredients

2 tbsps (melted) ghee

2 pounds (remove skin) chicken drumsticks

1/4 cup hot sauce

Method

1. Spread avocado oil into the basket of an air fryer. For 2-3 minutes, heat up air fryer to 400°F. Add drumsticks into the preheated air fryer and cook for 15 minutes. Turn chicken drumsticks and cook for 5 more minutes.

2. Add hot sauce and melted ghee into a big bowl and mix until combined. Add chicken drumsticks into the big bowl of sauce and toss until wholly coated. Move the coated chicken drumsticks into the air fryer basket and top with the remaining sauce.

3. Cook until an internal temperature of 165°F is reached, for 5 more minutes. Serve as desired.

Nutritional Information/Serving

Calories 983 kcal, Protein 110g, Carbs 5g, Fat 55g

Cheesy Turkey Wing

Preparation Time: 10 minutes

Cook Time: 15 minutes

Serves: 4 servings

Ingredients

½ cup parmesan cheese, grated

2 pounds (cut into drumettes and flats, and pat dry) turkey wings

1 teaspoon Herbes de Provence

1 teaspoon paprika

Avocado oil

Salt

Method

1. Add turkey wings into a bowl and let sit. Add salt, herbes de Provence, paprika, and parmesan into a small bowl and mix until combined. Add turkey wings into the cheese mixture until wholly coated. Heat up air fryer to 350°F.

2. Coat the wire basket of an air fryer with avocado oil. Work in batches, add turkey wings into the preheated air fryer, and cook for 15 minutes. Flip turkey wings midway while cooking. Serve garnished as desired with parmesan cheese.

Nutritional Information/Serving

Calories 633 kcal, Fat 38.4g, Protein 65.6g, Carb 2g

Delicious Turkey Drumsticks

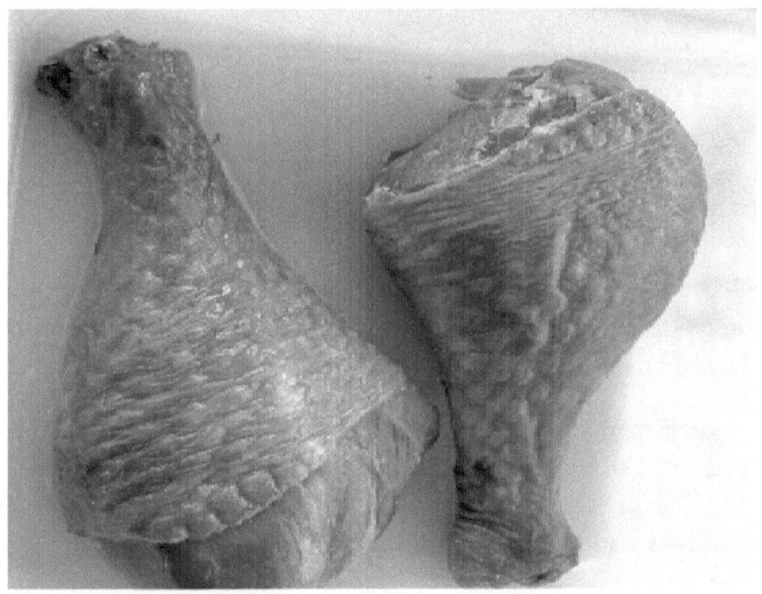

Preparation Time: 10 minutes

Cook Time: 20 minutes

Serves: 6 servings

Ingredients

1/4 cup coconut flour

2 1/2 pounds turkey drumsticks

1/4 tsp black pepper

1/2 tsp sea salt

1 cup pork rinds crumbs

2 eggs, large

1/2 teaspoon garlic powder

1 teaspoon paprika, smoked

1/4 teaspoon sage, dried

Method

1. Add black pepper, salt and coconut flour into an average flat-bottomed bowl, stir to combine and let sit. Crack the eggs into another bowl, whisk to combine and let sit. Add dried sage, garlic powder, smoked paprika and pork rind crumbs into another bowl and stir until combined.

2. Dip turkey drumsticks into the flour mixture until wholly coated. Immerse in the bowl with egg wash and shake to remove any excess. Press coated turkey pieces into the crumb mixture until combined.

3. For 5 minutes, heat up air fryer to 400°F. Coat the wired basket of the preheated air fryer lightly. Add breaded turkey onto the prepared air fryer basket in one layer, leaving enough room between each piece. Seal air fryer and cook until an internal temperature of 165°F is reached, for 20 minutes.

Nutritional Information/Serving

Calories 273 kcal, Net Carbs 2g, Protein 28g, Fat 15g

Delicious Turkey Tenders

Preparation Time: 10 minutes

Cook Time: 10 minutes

Serves: 2 servings

Ingredients

2 eggs

1 1/2 pounds (patted dry) turkey tenders

2 tbsp flax seed, ground

1 cup almond flour, fine

1 tsp sea salt, fine

1 tsp Italian seasoning

1/2 tsp black pepper, ground

1 tsp paprika

1/2 tsp onion powder

1/2 tsp garlic powder

Avocado oil cooking spray

Method

1. Heat up air fryer at 400°F. Sprinkle pepper and salt over pat dried turkey tenders to season. Add eggs into an average bowl and whisk. Add every seasoning, flaxseed and almond flour into a big flat-bottomed bowl and whisk mixture to combine.

2. Immerse the turkey tenders into the egg bowl and dip into the flour mixture until turkey is wholly coated. Spread avocado oil on the wired basket of the air fryer until liberally covered and top with turkey tenders, with enough room between each turkey tender.

3. Lightly coat turkey tenders with avocado oil. Air fry for 5 minutes, flip turkey tenders and air fry until cooked through, for 5 more minutes. Repeat process until no turkey tender remain uncooked.

Nutritional Information/Serving

Calories 315 kcal, Protein 17.2g, Carbs 12.9g, Fat 21.1g

Turkey Breast with Darkening Spice

Preparation Time: 10 minutes

Cook Time: 20 minutes

Serves: 2 servings

Ingredients

1 tsp oregano, ground

2 tsps paprika

½ tsp cayenne pepper

1 tsp cumin

½ tsp black pepper

½ tsp onion powder

2 tsps avocado oil

¼ tsp salt

2 (12 oz.) turkey breast halves, boneless skinless

Method

1. Add salt, black pepper, onion powder, cayenne pepper, cumin, oregano and paprika into a bowl and mix until combined. Pour the mixture into a platter. Coat each turkey breast with avocado oil until wholly covered.

2. Add each turkey breast into the plate with the spice mixture, roll and press until turkey is wholly coated. For 5 minutes, heat up air fryer to 360°F. Transfer the spice-coated turkey breasts into the wire basket of the preheated air fryer.

3. Cook turkey for 10 minutes before turning. Cook for 10 more minutes. Let turkey sit in a platter to cool for 5 minutes. Serve and dig in.

Nutritional Information/Serving

Calories 432 kcal, Protein 79.4g, Carbs 3.2g, Fat 9.5g

Crushed Turkey Tenderloins

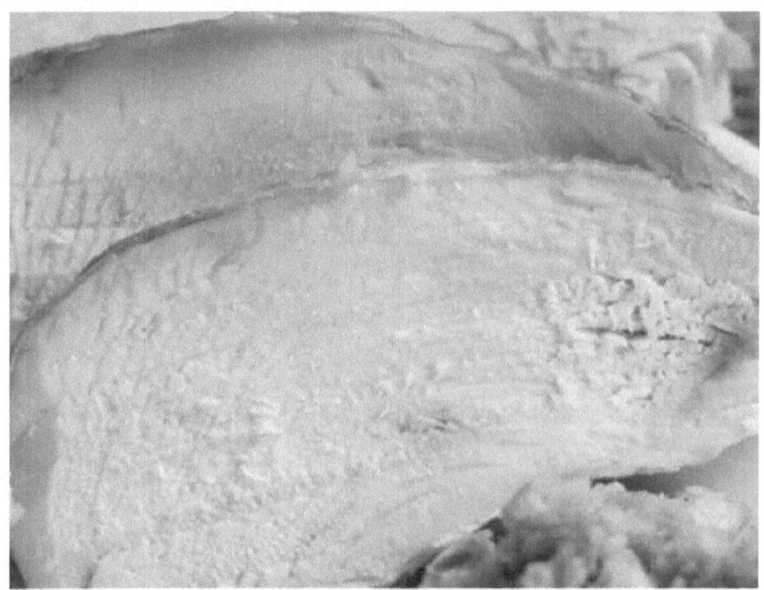

Preparation Time: 15 minutes

Cook Time: 12 minutes

Serves: 4 servings

Ingredients

½ cup crumbled pork rind

1 egg

8 turkey tenderloins

2 tbsps avocado oil

Method

1. Heat up air fryer to 350°F. Add egg into a bowl and beat. Add avocado oil and pork rind crumbs into a separate bowl and mix until combined. Immerse each turkey piece into the egg bowl and shake off any excess.

2. Transfer the turkey piece into the rind mixture until wholly coated. Transfer the breaded turkey into the wire basket of an air fryer. Cook for about 12 minutes, until an internal temperature of 165°F is reached and no pink remains in the middle.

Nutritional Information/Serving

Calories 159 kcal, Protein 18g, Carbs 0.1g, Fat 9.4g

Yummy Air Fried Turkey

Preparation Time: 10 minutes

Cook Time: 20 minutes

Serves: 10 servings

Ingredients

1 cup almond milk

5 lbs. turkey pieces

2 cups pork rinds, crushed

1 tbsp white vinegar

1/2 tsp rosemary

1/2 tsp salt

1/3 tsp cilantro

1/2 tsp mint

1 tsp black pepper

1 tsp celery salt

4 tsps paprika

1 tsp mustard, dried

1 tsp ginger, ground

2 tsps garlic salt

1 tbsp coconut oil

3 tsps white pepper

Method

1. Add vinegar and almond milk into a small bowl and mix. Add turkey pieces into a big bowl. Pour the vinegar-milk mixture over turkey until wholly coated. Refrigerate turkey mixture for 2 hours until marinated.

2. Add white pepper, ground ginger, garlic salt, paprika, dried mustard, black pepper, celery salt, cilantro, mint, rosemary, salt and pork rinds into a big flat-bottomed bowl and combine. Immerse turkey pieces in the rind mixture until wholly covered.

3. Sprinkle 1 tbsp coconut oil into the wire basket of the air fryer. Place turkey in one layer on the greased air fryer basket. Air fry turkey for 10 minutes at 360°F. Rotate air fryer basket and air fry until an internal temp of 165°F is reached, for 10 more minutes.

Nutritional Information/Serving

Calories 539 kcal, Fat 37g, Protein 45g, Carbs 1g

Air Fryer Turkey Nuggets with Sauce

Preparation Time: 10 minutes

Cook Time: 15 minutes

Serves: 4 servings

Ingredients

Avocado oil cooking spray

6 tablespoons sesame seeds, toasted

4 egg whites

1/2 teaspoon ground ginger

1/4 cup coconut flour

1 teaspoon sesame oil

1 pinch sea salt

1 lb. turkey breast, skinless boneless

Sauce

4 teaspoons coconut aminos

2 tablespoons almond butter

2 teaspoons rice vinegar

1 tablespoon water

1/2 teaspoon ginger, ground

1 teaspoon sriracha

1/2 teaspoon monk fruit

Method

1. Heat up air fryer for 10 minutes at 400°F. In the meantime, slice turkey into 1" nuggets and let sit in a bowl to dry. Sprinkle sesame oil and salt over turkey nuggets and toss until coated. Add ground ginger and coconut flour into a big zip-top bag and shake until combined.

2. Add the turkey into the bag mixture and shake until wholly coated. Add egg whites into a big bowl, add in the turkey pieces and toss until wholly covered with egg whites. Add in sesame seeds into a big zip-top bag. Shake off excess egg from the turkey nuggets and add into the bag with sesame seeds.

3. Shake turkey nuggets until well covered with sesame seeds. Spread avocado oil cooking spray on the wire basket of the air fryer until liberally covered. Add in the turkey nuggets. Note: avoid overcrowding. Lightly spread avocado oil over turkey nuggets.

4. Cook turkey nuggets for 6 minutes. Turn each turkey nugget, spray with avocado oil and cook until the outside is crisped and no pink remains internally, for 5-6 minutes. In the meantime, added every sauce ingredient into an average bowl and whisk until a smooth consistency is reached.

5. Serve turkey nuggets with the sauce.

Nutritional Information/Serving

Calories 286 kcal, Protein 29.9g, Carbs 10.3g, Fat 11.6g

SEAFOOD

Parchment-Paper Cod

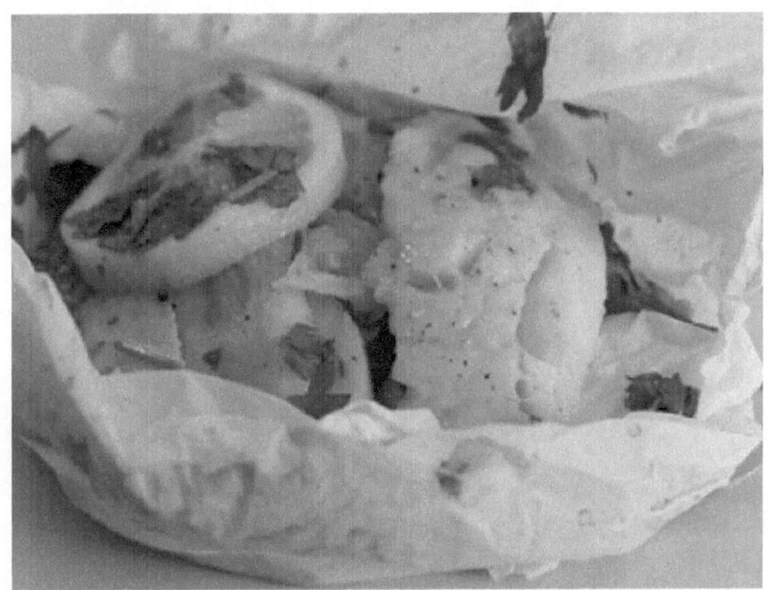

Preparation Time: 10 minutes

Cook Time: 15 minutes

Serves: 2 servings

Ingredients

1/2 cup carrots, julienned

2 (5 ounces) thawed cod fillets

1/2 cup red peppers, sliced thin

1/2 cup fennel bulbs, julienned

2 dollops butter, melted

2 dried thyme

1 tbsp (divided) salt

1 tbsp lime juice

1 tbsp avocado oil

1/2 tsp pepper

Method

1. Add lime juice, 1/2 tsp salt, thyme and melted butter into a fairly big bowl. Stir until a creamy and smooth consistency is reached. Add chopped veggies into the sauce and stir until combined.

2. Prepare 2 parchment paper squares big enough to hold veggies and fish. Spray avocado oil over fillet and season evenly with pepper and salt. Place a seasoned fillet on each parchment paper squash and top with even amount of sauce and veggies.

3. Fold paper over fish filling until enclosed like a packet and place in a fryer basket. Cook for 15 minutes at 350°. Open pack just before you serve and enjoy.

Nutritional Information/Serving

Calories 251 kcal, Protein 26g, Dietary Fiber 2g, Carbs 8g, Fat 12g

Cajun Halibut

Preparation Time: 10 minutes

Cook Time: 10 minutes

Serves: 2 servings

Ingredients

2 (6 oz.) {rinse and pat dry} halibut fillets, skin-on

1 tsp stevia powder

1 tbsp Cajun seasoning

2 tbsps avocado oil

Method

1. Heat up air fryer to 390°F. Coat the wire basket of an air fryer with cooking spray. Add stevia powder and Cajun seasoning into a small bowl and stir until combined.

2. Pour the stevia mixture into a platter. Add the fillets to the plate with seasoning until wholly coated on both sides. Transfer the halibut fillets into the prepared air fryer basket with the skin-side down.

3. Spray halibut with avocado oil. Seal the lid and cook for 8 minutes. Move out of the air fryer and let sit to cool for 2 minutes. Serve and enjoy.

Nutritional Information/Serving

Calories 253 kcal, Protein 30g, Carbs 0g, Fat 14.1g

Creamy Kale and Scallops

Preparation Time: 5 minutes

Cook Time: 10 minutes

Serves: 2 servings

Ingredients

1 tbsp tomato paste

3/4 cup heavy whipping cream

1 tsp garlic, minced

1 tbsp fresh chopped oregano

1/2 tsp ground black pepper

1/2 tsp salt

8 jumbo sea scallops

1 (12 ounces) (thaw and drain) kale, frozen

Sea and pepper, to taste

Avocado oil

Method

1. Coat a 7" baking pan with avocado oil. Add in the kale in a single layer at the base of the prepared baking pan. Evenly coat scallops with avocado oil and season with pepper and salt.

2. Transfer seasoned scallops into the baking pan over the kale. Add pepper, salt, garlic, oregano, tomato paste and heavy whipping cream into a small bowl and mix until combined.

3. Pour cream mixture over mixture in the baking pan. Transfer pan into the wire basket of the air fryer, and cook until sauce is bubbly and hot, and scallops is well cooked, for 10 minutes at 350°F.

4. Serve and enjoy.

Nutritional Information/Serving

Calories 359 kcal, Fat 33g, Protein 9g, Carbs 6g

Cheesy Shrimp with Herbs

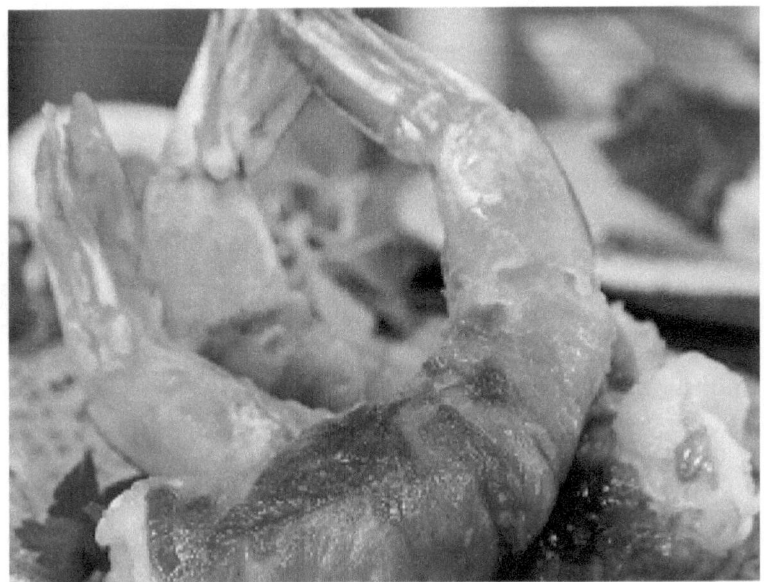

Preparation Time: 5 minutes

Cook Time: 10 minutes

Serves: 6 servings

Ingredients

4 minced garlic cloves

2 lbs. (peeled and deveined) cooked shrimp, jumbo

1 tsp pepper

2/3 cup grated parmesan cheese

1 tsp chives

1/2 tsp tarragon

2 tbsps avocado oil

1 tsp onion powder

Lime, quartered

Method

1. Add avocado oil, onion powder, chives, tarragon, pepper, parmesan cheese and garlic into a big bowl and combine. Add in the shrimp and toss lightly until wholly coated. Spread avocado oil over the basket of the air fryer.

2. Add in the coated shrimp and cook until the coating on shrimp is browned, for 8-10 minutes at 350°F. Serve shrimp, topped with lime juice.

Nutritional Information/Serving

Calories 201 kcal, Protein 23.5g, Carbs 4.8g, Fat 8.9g

Fried Shrimp Scampi

Preparation Time: 5 minutes

Cook Time: 10 minutes

Serves: 4 servings

Ingredients

1 tbsp lime juice

4 tbsps butter

2 tsps red pepper flakes

1 tbsp garlic, minced

1 tbsp fresh copped oregano

1 tbsp chopped sage

1 pound shrimp, thaw

2 tbsps chicken stock

Method

1. Heat up air fryer to 330ºF. Add a 3-by-6" baking pan into the wire basket of the preheating air fryer and let sit until heated. Add red pepper flakes, garlic and butter into the heated pan, stir and air fry until the garlic is infused and butter is melted, for 2 minutes.

2. Add every other ingredient into the pan and stir lightly. Seal the air fryer and air fry for 5 minutes. Stir the shrimp once while cooking. Carefully take out pan from the air fryer, stir shrimp mixture again and let sit for a minute.

3. Stir one more time and season with any remaining fresh chopped oregano.

Nutritional Information/Serving

Calories 221 kcal, Fat 13g, Protein 23g, Carbs 1g

Lime Trout Patties

Preparation Time: 5 minutes

Cook Time: 7 minutes

Serves: 2 servings

Ingredients

1 (beaten) eggs

8 ounces (minced) fresh trout fillet

1/4 tsp garlic powder

1/8 tsp salt

1 lime, sliced

Method

1. Add every ingredient into a bowl, excluding the limes. Mold mixture into small patties. Heat up air fryer to 390°F. Add lime slices into the basket of an air fryer and top with the salmon patties. Cook at 390°F for 7 minutes.

2. Let sit to cool slightly and serve as desired.

Nutritional Information/Serving

Calories 197 kcal, Protein 25.9g, Carbs 0.5g, Fat 9.2g

Crispy Catfish Sticks

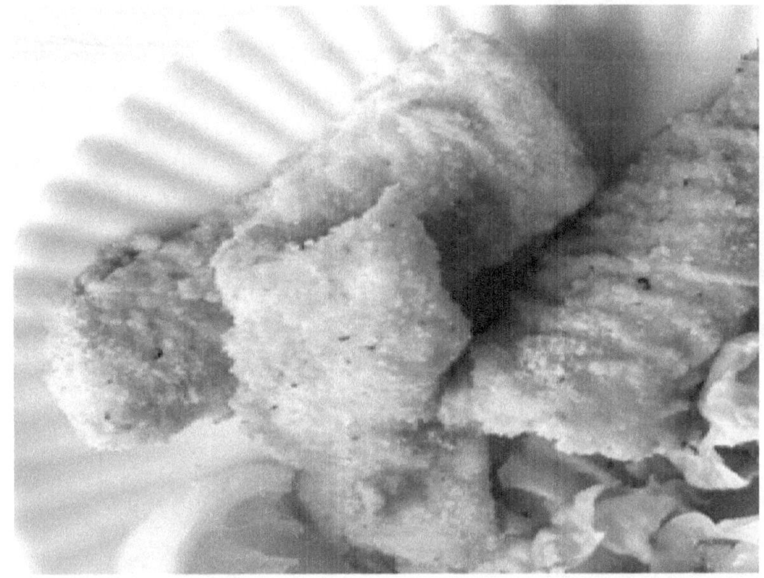

Preparation Time: 10 minutes

Cook Time: 10 minutes

Serves: 4 servings

Ingredients

1/4 cup mayo

1 pound (pat dry and slice into sticks) catfish

2 tablespoons water

2 tablespoons Dijon mustard

3/4 teaspoon Cajun seasoning

1 1/2 cups pork rind, crumbled

Salt and pepper, as necessary

Method

1. Coat the wire basket of an air fryer with avocado oil. Add water, mustard and mayonnaise into a small flat-bottomed bowl, and whisk until combined. Add Cajun seasoning, pork rind crumbs, pepper and salt into a second flat-bottomed bowl and whisk until combined.

2. Dip each fish stick into the mustard-mayo mixture and shake off excess. Immerse fish stick into the crumb mixture and toss until coated. Repeat process with the remaining fish sticks.

3. Add breaded fish sticks into the prepared air fryer basket and cook for 10 minutes at 400°F. Flip fish sticks over midway during cooking. Serve at once.

Nutritional Information/Serving

Calories 263 kcal, Protein 26.3g, Carbs 1g, Fat 16g

Air Fryer Coconut Shrimp

Preparation Time: 10 minutes

Cook Time: 15 minutes

Serves: 4 servings

Ingredients

1 teaspoon salt

1/4 cup almond flour

1 cup sweetened coconut flakes

2 egg whites

1/2 lb. large raw shrimp

2 tbsps avocado oil

Method

1. Add coconut flakes into a flat-bottomed bowl. Add egg whites into a separate flat-bottomed bowl. Add salt and almond flour into third flat-bottomed bowl and combine. Dip a shrimp into the flour mixture until coated. Dip into the egg whites and immerse in the coconut flakes.

2. Add breaded shrimp into platter and repeat process with the remaining shrimps. Coat the wired basket of an air fryer with avocado oil. Working in batches, add the breaded shrimp into the prepared air fryer and cook for 10-15 minutes at 330°F.

3. Serve as desired.

Nutritional Information/Serving

Calories 214 kcal, Protein 11.7g, Total Carbs 15.4g, Fat 18g

Yummy Avocado Halibut Cakes

Preparation Time: 15 minutes

Cook Time: 15 minutes

Serves: 4 servings

Ingredients

1/4 cup mashed avocado

1 pound fresh Alaskan halibut side, skinless

1 1/2 teaspoon curry powder, yellow

1/4 cup chopped parsley

1/4 cup (divided) coconut flour + 2 teaspoons

1/2 teaspoon sea salt

1/2 cup coconut flakes

2 (whisked) eggs

Melted coconut oil

Greens

6 cups (tightly packed) spinach and arugula mix

2 teaspoons melted coconut oil

1 pinch sea salt

Method

1. Chop the halibut and transfer into a big bowl. Add salt, curry powder, parsley and avocado into the big bowl and stir until combined. Add in the 2 teaspoons coconut flour into the bowl and combine. Prepare a parchment paper lined baking sheet. Form halibut into 8 (1/4 cup) sized patties.

2. Add halibut patties onto the prepared baking sheet, and transfer into a freezer for 20 minutes. In the meantime, heat up air fryer for 10 minutes at 400°F. Coat air fryer basket with melted coconut oil.

3. Add the coconut flakes, 1/4 cup coconut flour and the whisked eggs into 3 individual shallow dishes. Immerse the chilled patties into the coconut flour until wholly coated and move into the egg wash until wholly coated. Brush off excess egg and press a side of the halibut patties into coconut flakes until covered.

4. Place halibut cakes into the wired basket of an air fryer, with the flaky side on top. Lightly brush halibut cakes with melted coconut oil and cook for about 15 minutes, until soft and juicy internally, and crisped and golden brown externally. Use a spatula to remove cooked halibut cakes.

5. Add coconut oil into a big skillet over med-heat. Add in the veggie mix into the pan and season with salt. Stir cook for 30-60 seconds, until just wilted. Split cooked greens into platters, topped with halibut cakes.

Nutritional Information/Serving

Calories 519 kcal, Protein 41.2g, Carbs 22.7g, Fat 29g

Air Fryer Trout with Lime Wedges

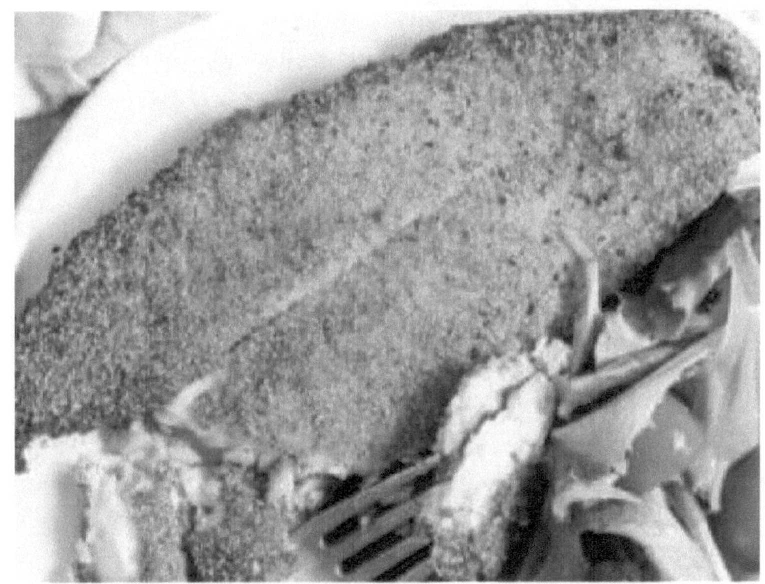

Preparation Time: 10 minutes

Cook Time: 7 minutes

Serves: 2 servings

Ingredients

2 teaspoons avocado oil

2 (even thickness) trout fillets, at room temp

Coarse black pepper and salt, to taste

2 teaspoons paprika

Lime wedges

Method

1. Coat trout fillets with avocado oil until wholly covered and season with pepper, salt and paprika. Transfer fillets into an air fryer basket. Seal the lid and cook for 7 minutes at 390°F.

2. Check for doneness, by flaking fish with a fork. Let sit to cool, serve and enjoy.

Nutritional Information/Serving

Calories 288 kcal, Protein 28.3g, Carbs 1.4g, Fat 18.9g

Lemon Shrimp Skewers

Preparation Time: 5 minutes

Cook Time: 8 minutes

Serves: 2 servings

Ingredients

1 garlic clove

1 cup (thaw) shrimp, raw

1/8 tsp salt

1 lemon

5 (6") bamboo skewers, soak for 20 minutes in water

Freshly ground pepper, to taste

Method

1. Heat up air fryer to 350°F. Add minced garlic, lemon juice and shrimp into a bowl and mix until combined. Sprinkle with pepper and salt. Thread shrimp on the skewers and transfer into the wire basket of the preheated air fryer.

2. Cook for 4 minutes. Flip shrimp skewers and cook for 4 more minutes. Sprinkle with fresh chopped parsley and serve.

Nutritional Information/Serving

Calories 62 kcal, Protein 12.3g, Carbs 1g, Fat 1g

Asparagus Halibut

Preparation Time: 5 minutes

Cook Time: 8 minutes

Serves: 2 servings

Ingredients

1 tbsp avocado oil

1 1/2 tbsps lime juice

2 tbsps fresh chopped cilantro

2 tbsps (chopped coarsely) fresh sage

1 (450g) bunch asparagus

2 (6 oz ea) fresh halibut fillets

salt and pepper, to taste

Method

1. Add pepper, salt, cilantro, sage, avocado oil and lime juice into a small bowl and mix until combined. Spread 3/4 of the herb mixture over fillets until wholly coated.

2. Add the remaining herb mixture and the asparagus into an average bowl and combine thoroughly. Evenly spread asparagus mixture in the basket of an air fryer. Add the halibut fillets over asparagus layer.

3. Seal the air fryer lid and cook until desired doneness is reached, for 6-8 minutes at 400°F. Serve, topped with lime juice and dig in.

Nutritional Information/Serving

Calories 391 kcal, Protein 48g, Carbs 9g, Fat 19g

Air Fried Flounder Sticks

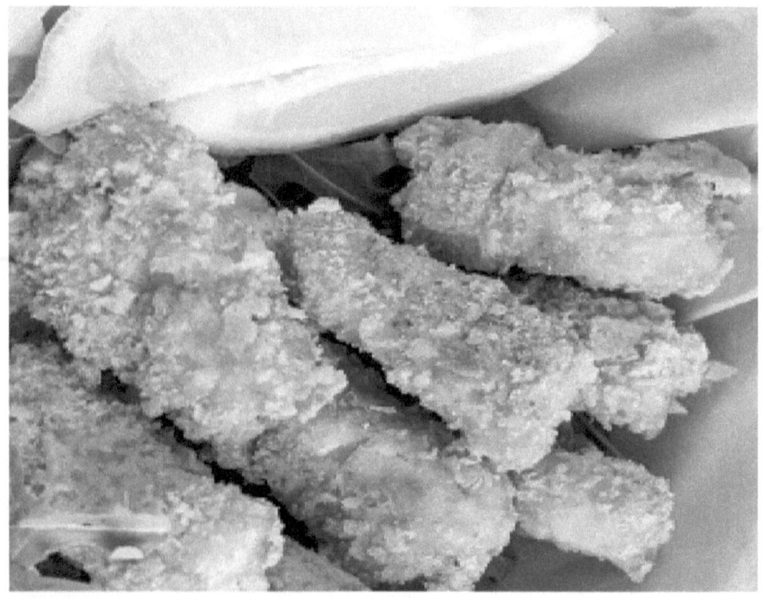

Preparation Time: 10 minutes

Cook Time: 10 minutes

Serves: 4 servings

Ingredients

1/4 cup mayo

1 pound (pat dry and slice into 1-by-2" wide sticks) flounder

2 tablespoons water

2 tablespoons Dijon mustard

3/4 teaspoon Cajun seasoning

1 1/2 cups pork rind

Salt and pepper, as necessary

Method

1. Coat the wired basket of an air fryer with avocado oil. Add water, mustard and mayonnaise into a small flat-bottomed bowl and whisk until combined. Add Cajun seasoning and pork rinds into a second flat-bottomed bowl and whisk to combine.

2. Sprinkle pepper and salt over pork rind mixture to taste. Immerse fish sticks into the mustard mixture until coated and shake off any excess. Immerse the coated sticks into the pork rind mixture and toss until wholly coated.

3. Transfer the fish sticks to the prepared air fryer basket. Cook for 5 minutes at 400°F. Use tong to turn the fish sticks and cook for 5 more minutes. Serve at once.

Nutritional Information/Serving

Calories 263 kcal, Protein 26.4g, Carbs 1g, Fat 16g

Yummy Breaded Shrimp

Preparation Time: 10 minutes

Cook Time: 6 minutes

Serves: 3 servings

Ingredients

¾ cup coconut flour

1 lb. (peel and clean) shrimp

1 tsp garlic powder

1 tsp onion powder

½ cup pork rind crumbs

2 (beaten lightly) eggs

Salt & fresh pepper

1/2 cup shredded coconut flakes, unsweetened

½ cup mayonnaise, full fat

Avocado oil

1 (grate finely) garlic clove

1/2 lemon, juiced and zested

2-3 tbsps sriracha

Method

1. Add few cracks of pepper, 1/2 tsp salt, 1 tsp garlic powder, 1 tsp onion powder and coconut flakes into a flat-bottomed dish and mix until well combined. Add eggs into a small bowl and whisk until lightly beaten.

2. Add pork rind crumbs into then coconut flakes mixture and stir until well combined. Sprinkle a small pinch of salt over shrimp until evenly seasoned. Immerse shrimp in coconut flour until coated and shake off excess. Dip in the eggs and shake off excess. Immerse in the rind mixture until wholly coated.

3. Coat the wire basket of an air fryer with avocado oil. Work in batches, add the coasted shrimp into the prepared air fryer basket and cook at 390°F for 4 minutes. Flip and cook for 4 more minutes. Repeat process with remaining shrimp. Serve and dig in.

Nutritional Information/Shrimp

Calories 75 kcal, Protein 3.2g, Protein 3.2g, Fat 4g, Carbs 2g

Scallop with Bacon Wraps

Preparation Time: 15 minutes

Cook Time: 20 minutes

Serves: 9 servings

Ingredients

2 tbsps Sriracha sauce

1/2 cup mayo

1 pinch coarse salt

1 lb. (pat dry with paper towel) bay scallops

12 (cut into third) bacon slices

1 pinch black pepper, freshly cracked

Avocado oil

Method

1. Add sriracha sauce and mayo into a small bowl and mix until combined. Place mayonnaise mixture in the refrigerator to chill. Heat up air fryer to 390°F. Sprinkle pepper and salt over scallops.

2. Wrap 1/3 of a bacon slice over each scallop and hold in place with a toothpick. Coat the wire basket of the preheated air fryer with avocado oil. Work in batches, add the scallop wraps in the air fryer basket in one layer.

3. Cook until crisped and opaque, for 7 minutes. Check doneness; if necessary, cook for 1-2 more minutes until desired doneness is reached.

Transfer the cooked scallops onto a plate lined with paper towel and serve with the chilled mayo sauce.

Nutritional Information/Serving

Calories 222 kcal, Protein 17.3g, Carbs 3.3g, Fat 15.3g

Crab Patties

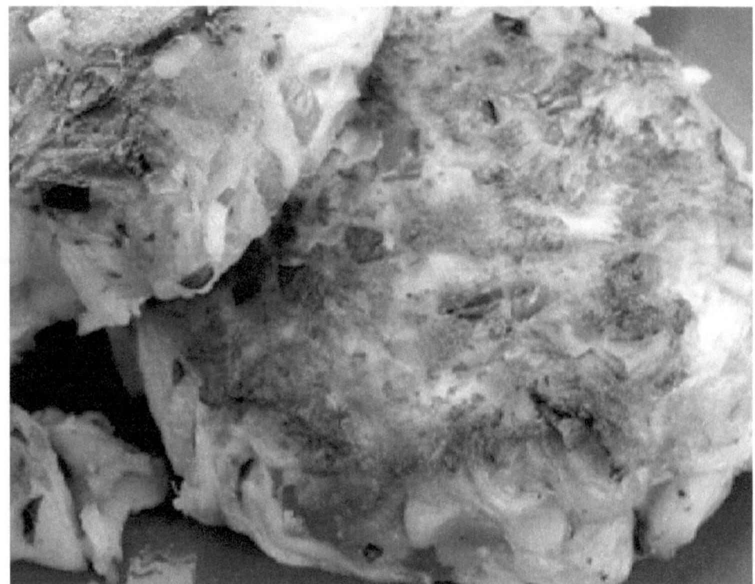

Preparation Time: 10 minutes

Cook Time: 15 minutes

Serves: 3 servings

Ingredients

1/4 cup mayo

3/4 cup crumbled pork rind

2 tsps Worcestershire sauce

1 egg

3/4 tsp Cajun seasoning

1 tsp Dijon mustard

1/4 tsp cayenne pepper

1/2 tsp salt

4 oz. lump crabmeat, fresh

1/4 tsp white pepper, ground

Method

1. Heat up air fryer to 370°F. Add pepper, cayenne, salt, Cajun seasoning, mustard, Worcestershire sauce, egg, mayo and pork rind crumbs into a small bowl and mix until combined. Lightly fold in the crab meat into the pork rind mixture.

2. Shape mixture into 3 even crab patties and transfer onto a round parchment paper sheet. Place parchment sheet in the wire basket of the preheated air fryer. Cook crab patties for 6 minutes before turning. Cook for 6 more minutes, until patties are browned.

3. Serve as desired and dig in.

Nutritional Information/Serving

Calories 274 kcal, Protein 19g, Carbs 1.2g, Fat 21.3g

Butter Sauced Halibut

Preparation Time: 5 minutes

Cook Time: 15 minutes

Serves: 4 servings

Ingredients

Salt and ground black pepper to taste

4 (6 oz.) halibut fillets

2/3 cup butter

Avocado oil spray

Method

1. Heat up air fryer to 350°F. Sprinkle pepper and salt over halibut fillets and mist with avocado oil until evenly coated. Transfer the seasoned halibut fillets into the wire basket of the preheated air fryer in a single layer.

2. Cook halibut fillets for 12 minutes, until fish has a golden hue and is easily flaked with a fork. In the meantime, add butter into a small deep skillet over med-low heat and bring to simmering. Cook for 3-5 minutes, until butter is brown and frothy.

3. Serve cooked halibut fillets with Browned butter.

Nutritional Information/Serving

Calories 416 kcal, Protein 31.8g, Carbs 0g, Fat 31.9g

APPETIZERS

Crunchy Avocado Fries

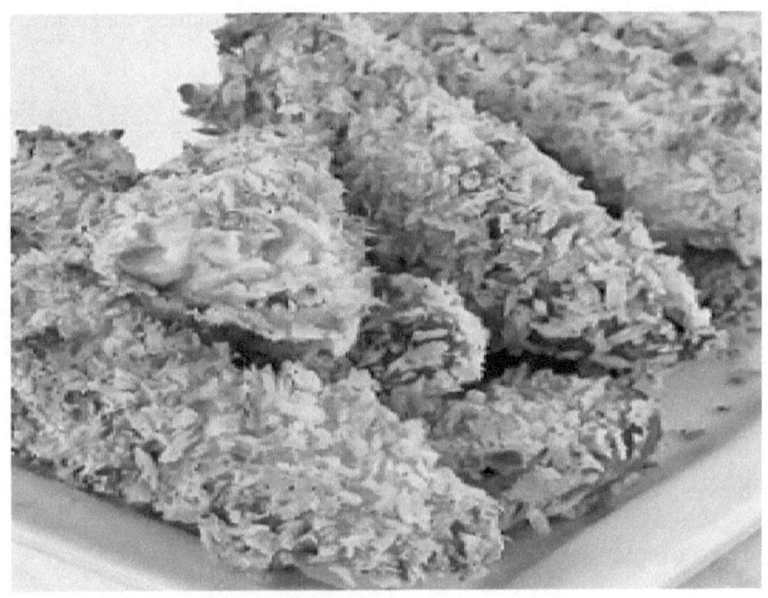

Preparation Time: 10 minutes

Cook Time: 10 minutes

Serves: 2 servings

Ingredients

1 egg

1 (halved, pitted and cut into wedges) avocado, ripe but firm

1/2 tsp salt

1/2 cup pork rind crumbs

Method

1. Add salt and egg into a bowl and beat together. Add pork rind crumbs into a separate bowl. Immerse avocado wedges in the egg wash and transfer into the bowl with pork rind. Heat up air fryer to 400°F.

2. Add the breaded avocados into the wire basket of the preheated air fryer in one layer. Cook until well cooked, for 8-10 minutes. Shake air fryer basket midway while cooking.

Nutritional Information/Serving

Calories 196 kcal, Protein 9.5g, Total Carbs 6.2g, Fat 15.4g

Cauli-Nuggets

Preparation Time: 5 minutes

Cook Time: 10 minutes

Serves: 4 servings

Ingredients

1 cup pork rind crumbs

1 egg

1/2 tsp salt

1/2 head (cut into florets) cauliflower

Freshly ground black pepper

1/2 tsp garlic powder

1/2 cup hot sauce

1 cup ranch dressing

Method

1. Add pepper, garlic powder, salt, and egg into a bowl and mix until combined. Add pork rind crumbs into a separate bowl. Heat up air fryer to 400°F. Immerse cauliflower florets into the egg wash and transfer into the bowl with pork rind crumbs.

2. Add the breaded cauliflower into the air fryer basket and cook for 4-5 minutes. Shake basket and cook until well cooked, for 4-5 more minutes. In the meantime, add hot sauce and ranch dressing into a bowl and combine.

3. Serve cauli-nuggets with hot ranch sauce.

Nutritional Information/Serving

Calories 391 kcal, Protein 9.9g, Carbs 13.4g, Fat 32.1g

Bacon-Asparagus Wraps

Preparation Time: 5 minutes

Cook Time: 20 minutes

Serves: 6 servings

Ingredients

1 lb. (trim off ends) asparagus

1 lb. (halved) bacon

Creole seasoning, to taste

Salt and pepper, to taste

1 tablespoon avocado oil

Method

1. Add trimmed asparagus into a bowl and coat with avocado oil. Sprinkle creole seasoning, pepper and salt over coated asparagus and toss until

wholly coated. Wrap 2 asparagus spears in 1/2 bacon slice and transfer into the wire basket of the air fryer.

2. Cook until desired crispiness is reached, for 20 minutes. Flip bacon wrapped asparagus midway during cooking. Serve at once or transfer into well lidded containers and store for up to 7 days.

Nutritional Information/Serving

Calories 350 kcal, Fat 32g, Protein 11g, Carbs 3g

Fried Garlic

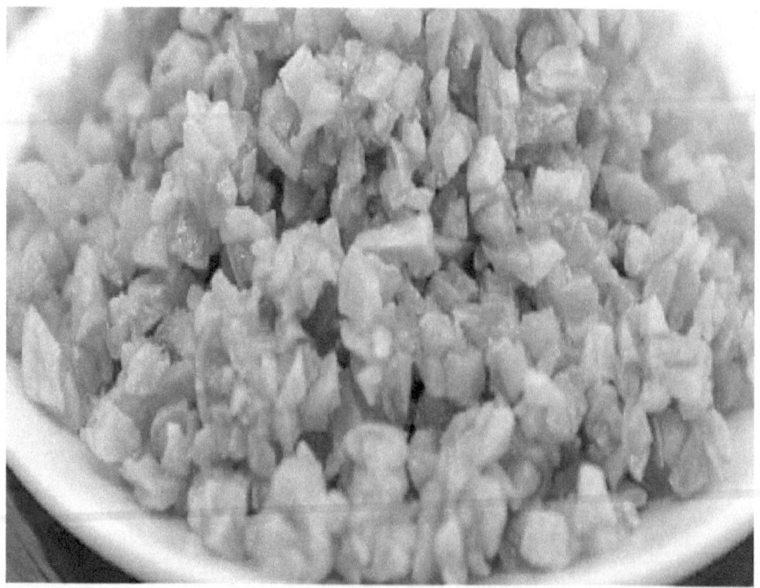

Preparation Time: 5 minutes

Cook Time: 20 minutes

Serves: 4 servings

Ingredients

2 tbsps avocado oil

1 (medium-sized) head garlic

Method

1. Slice 1/4" off the top of the garlic head. Dribble avocado oil over bare part of the garlic cloves and wrap tightly in foil. Add the wrapped garlic into a wire basket of an air fryer and cook for 20 minutes at 400°F. Check for softness and doneness.

2. Cook for 5-10 more minutes until well cooked. Let sit to cool before you serve.

Nutritional Information/Serving

Calories 89 kcal, Protein 0.8g, Carbs 4.5g, Fat 8.2g

Scotch Eggs

Preparation Time: 20 minutes

Cook Time: 25 minutes

Serves: 4 servings

Ingredients

1 tbsp (chop finely) sage

1 lb. pork sausage

1/8 tsp nutmeg, grated

2 tbsps fresh chopped cilantro

1/8 tsp ground black pepper

1/8 tsp salt

1 cup parmesan cheese, shredded

4 (peeled) eggs, hardboiled

2 tsps mustard, coarse-ground

Method

1. Add black pepper, salt, nutmeg, cilantro, sage, mustard and sausage into a big bowl and lightly mix until combined. Form mixture into 4 even patties. Place an egg on each patty and form patty around the egg. Repeat process with the remaining patties and eggs.

2. Immerse each egg and patty in shredded parmesan cheese, gently press and roll until wholly covered. Transfer eggs in the wire basket of an air fryer and coat lightly with avocado oil.

3. Cook scotch eggs for 15 minutes at 400°F. Flip eggs midway through air fryer and coat with avocado oil. Serve scotch eggs with mustard.

Nutritional Information/Serving

Calories 533 kcal, Fat 43g, Protein 33g, Carbs 2g

Romano Zucchini Fries

Preparation Time: 5 minutes

Cook Time: 10 minutes

Serves: 4 servings

Ingredients

1 (beaten) egg, large

2 (sliced into 1/2-by-3" sticks) zucchini, medium

½ cup (grated) pecorino romano cheese

½ cup almond flour

1 pinch pepper and salt

1 tsp Italian seasoning

Avocado oil

Method

1. Add pepper, salt, seasoning, grated pecorino romano cheese and almond flour into a flat-bottomed bowl and stir until well combined. Dip zucchini stick into the bowl with the beaten egg until wholly coated. Immerse coated zucchini into the cheese-flour mixture until wholly coated.

2. Transfer the coated zucchini sticks onto a platter and repeat process with the remaining zucchini sticks. Work in batches, coat the wired basket of the air fryer with avocado oil. Add zucchini sticks into the air fryer basket in one layer.

3. Seal the lid and cook until crisped, at 400°F for 10 minutes. Let sit to cool, serve and dig in.

Nutritional Information/Serving

Calories 147 kcal, Fat 10g, Fat 9g, Carbs 6g

Buffalo Cauli-Tots with Turkey

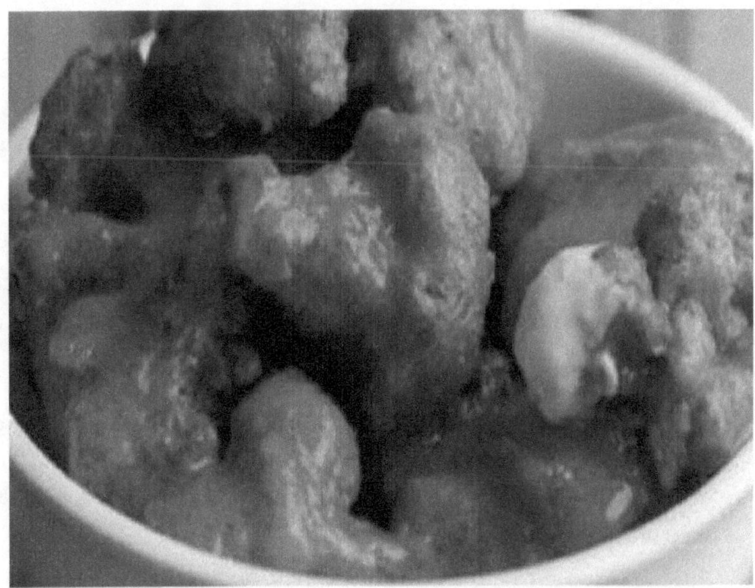

Preparation Time: 10 minutes

Cook Time: 5 minutes

Serves: 4 servings

Ingredients

1/2 tsp garlic powder

2 cups cauliflower florets

1 egg

8 oz. seasoned rotisserie turkey breast

2 tbsps buffalo sauce

3/4 cup parmesan cheese

Breading

4 tbsps parmesan cheese

6 tbsps almond flour

Method

1. Add buffalo sauce, 3/4 cup parmesan cheese, egg, garlic powder, turkey breast and cauliflower florets into a big bowl and combine well. Form mixture into 1 tsp-sized balls.

2. Heat up air fryer to 400°F. Add 6 tbsps almond flour and 4 tbsps parmesan cheese into a second bowl and stir until combined. Roll cauli-balls into the parmesan mixture until wholly coated and shape into cauli-tot shapes.

3. Coat the wire basket of an air fryer with avocado oil until evenly covered. Work in batches, add in the cauli-turkey tots in one layer, seal the lid and air fry for 6 minutes. Flip the tots and cook for 3 more minutes, until well cooked and browned.

4. Repeat process until cauli-turkey tots are well cooked and browned.

Nutritional Information/Serving

Calories 49 kcal, Protein 3g, Carbs 1g, Fat 3g

Cream Filled Jalapeno Poppers

Preparation Time: 10 minutes

Cook Time: 5 minutes

Serves: 5 servings

Ingredients

6 ounces cream cheese

10 (halved vertically and remove seeds) jalapenos

2 (cooked and crumbled) bacon slices

1/4 cup cheddar cheese, shredded

Avocado oil cooking spray

Method

1. Add cream cheese into a microwave-safe bowl and heat until softened, for 15 seconds in a microwave. Add shredded cheese, crumbled bacon and cream cheese into a bowl and mix until combined. Fill the poppers with the bacon mixture.

2. Add the filled jalapeño into the wired basket of the air fryer and cover evenly with avocado oil. Seal the lid and cook until desired tenderness is reached, for 5-7 minutes at 370°F. Let poppers sit to cool before you serve.

Nutritional Information/Serving

Calories 62 kcal, Fat 4g, Protein 3g, Carbs 3g

Air Fryer Pickles with Herbed Sauce

Preparation Time: 10 minutes

Cook Time: 10 minutes

Serves: 12 servings

Ingredients

1 cup coconut flour

12 (halved lengthways and pat dry lightly) pickle spears

2 eggs, large

2 1/2 oz. pkg. pork rinds, crumbled

Tarragon Sauce

1/2 tbsp tarragon, dried

8 oz. sour cream

1 tsps garlic powder

1 tsp vinegar

1/2 tsp salt

1/4 tsp pepper

Method

1. Add pork rinds into flat-bottomed bowl. Add eggs into a small bowl and whisk until beaten. Add coconut flour into a third bowl. Dip pickle pieces in the coconut flour until coated. Immerse in the egg wash and transfer into the bowl with pork rind until wholly coated.

2. Place breaded pickles in the wire basket of the air fryer and cook at 400°F for 7 minutes. Add every sauce ingredient in a bowl and whisk to combine. Serve fried pickles with herb sauce.

Nutritional Information/Serving

Calories 126 kcal, Fat 7g, Protein 6g, Carbs 7g

Asian Kkwari-Gochu

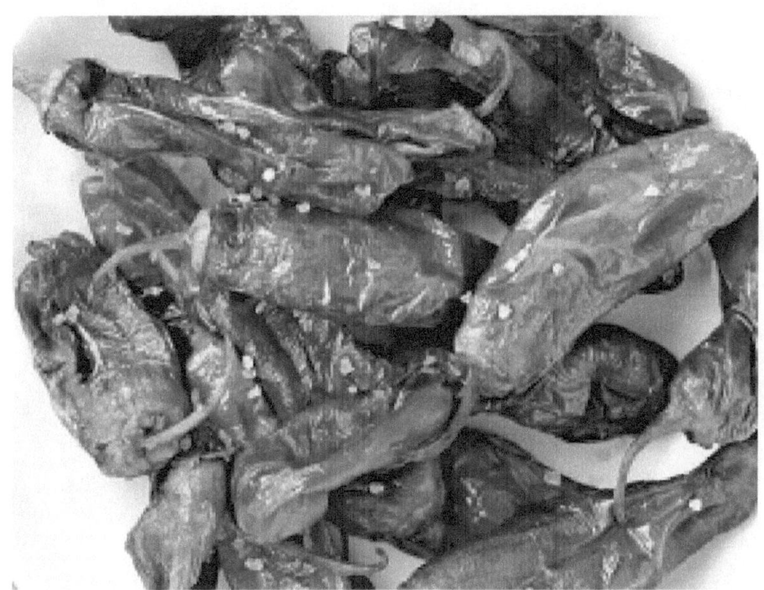

Preparation Time: 5 minutes

Cook Time: 10 minutes

Serves: 4 servings

Ingredients

Salt and pepper, as necessary

1 (6 ounces) bag shishito peppers, wash and pat dry.

1/3 cup finely grated parmesan cheese

1/2 tablespoons olive oil

1 Lemon, juiced

Method

1. Add the cleaned shishito peppers into a bowl and toss with pepper, salt, and olive oil until wholly coated. Transfer peppers into the wire basket of an air fryer and cook until blistered for 10 minutes at 350°F. Note: check every now and then to prevent burning.

2. Serve peppers, topped with grated parmesan cheese and lemon juice.

Nutritional Information/Serving

Calories 65 kcal, Protein 3.1g, Net Carb 1g, Fiber 1.5g, Fat 4g

Yummy Chicken Wings

Preparation Time: 5 minutes

Cook Time: 30 minutes

Serves: 3 servings

Ingredients

1/4 cup coconut oil

1 1/2 lbs. (cut at the joints with a big knife) chicken wings

1/4 cup hot sauce

Serve with

Ranch dip

Celery sticks

Method

1. Add chicken wings in the wire basket of an air fryer and cook for 15-20 minutes at 390°F. Flip the chicken wings over and cook until crisped and golden brown, for 10-15 more minutes.

2. Add coconut oil into the skillet over med-heat and melt. Add hot sauce into the coconut oil and stir until combined. Dribble sauce over chicken wings and toss until coated.

Nutritional Information/Serving

Calories 405 kcal, Fat 35g, Protein 23g, Carbs 1g

3-Cheese Filled Mushrooms

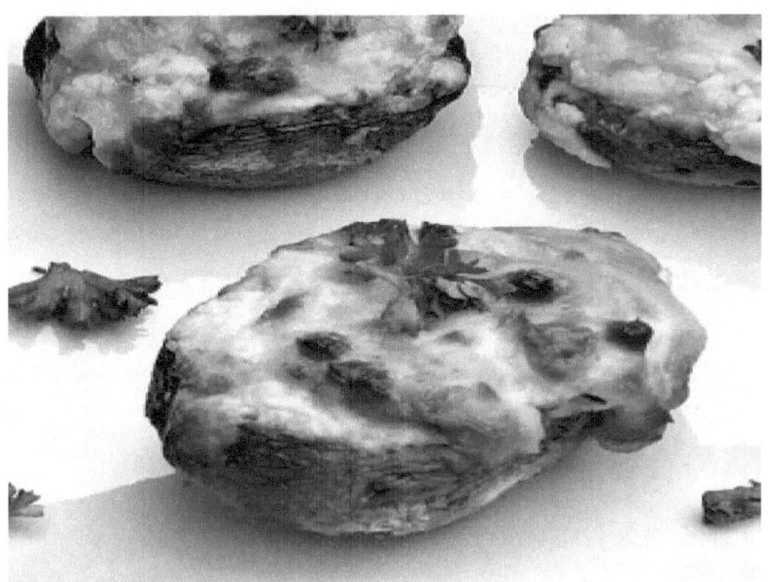

Preparation Time: 5 minutes

Cook Time: 8 minutes

Serves: 5 servings

Ingredients

4 ounces (reduced-fat) cream cheese

8 ounces (remove stems and chop into small pieces) fresh mushrooms, large

1/8 cup (shredded) sharp cheddar cheese

¼ cup (shredded) parmesan cheese

1 tsp Worcestershire sauce

1/8 cup (shredded) white cheddar cheese

Salt and pepper, as necessary

2 (chopped) garlic cloves

Method

1. Scoop out mushroom flesh from the place where stem stood until a large cavity is made. Add cream cheese into a heatproof bowl, place in a microwave and heat until tenderized, for 15 seconds.

2. Add Worcestershire sauce, pepper, salt, every shredded cheese and the melted cream cheese into an average bowl and mix until combined. Fill the mushroom holes with the cream cheese filling.

3. Transfer the stuffed mushrooms into the wire basket of an air fryer and cook at 370°F for 8 minutes. Let the stuffed mushrooms sit until cooled before you serve.

Nutritional Information/Serving

Calories 196 kcal, Protein 5.4g, Carbs 5.9g, Fat 18.3g

Roasted Pork Scratching

Preparation Time: 5 minutes

Cook Time: 15 minutes

Serves: 1 serving

Ingredients

300g pork rind, whole

Method

1. On a platter, add the pork rind with the skin side up and spread out. Place platter with the spread pork rind into a refrigerator for 24 hours until dried out.

2. Transfer pork rind onto the wire basket of an air fryer and cook plaint, for 4 minutes at 446°F. Slice pork rind into small pieces with a kitchen scissors, and return into the air fryer basket.

3. Cook until crackled, for 5 more minutes. Leave uncrackled pork rinds in the air fryer basket and move crackled pork pieces onto a plate lined with paper towel to drain.

4. Cook for 2 more minutes and repeat process in step 3 above, removing crackled pork pieces to the plate and leaving the uncrackled ones in the air fryer. Repeat process until pork rinds are fully crackled.

Nutritional Information/Serving

Calories 1675 kcal, Fat 131.5g, Protein 107.5g, Carbs 0.6g

Spicy Bacon Nuggets

Preparation Time: 5 minutes

Cook Time: 10 minutes

Serves: 4 servings

Ingredients

1/4 cup hot sauce

4 (slice into 6 equal pieces ea) bacon strips

1/2 cup pork rinds, crushed

Method

1. Add bacon bits into a bowl and top with hot sauce until wholly coated. Pour pork rind crumbs into a flat-bottomed bowl. Immerse bacon bits into rind until wholly coated. Transfer bacon bits into the wire basket of an air fryer. Seal the lid and cook for 8-10 minutes at 350°F.

Note: Check every now and then to prevent burning.

Nutritional Information/Serving

Calories 121 kcal, Protein 7.3g Carbs 0g, Fat 8.7g

Crisped Onion Rings

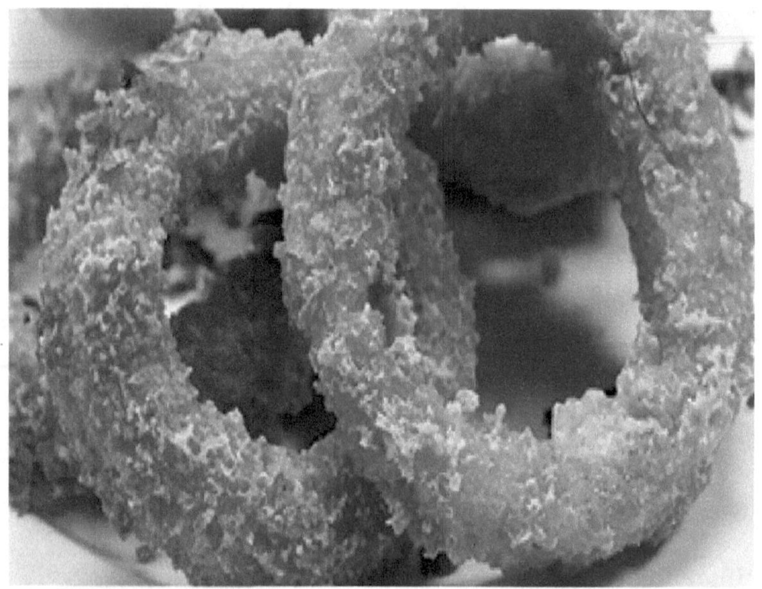

Preparation Time: 10 minutes

Cook Time: 20 minutes

Serves: 6 (3 onion rings) servings

Ingredients

2 eggs

1 (peeled and cut into 1/2" thick rings) yellow onion, large

1/4 cup ground flax seed

3/4 cup almond flour

1/4 teaspoon garlic powder

1/4 teaspoon paprika

1/4 teaspoon black pepper, ground

1/2 teaspoon salt

Avocado oil

Method

1. Coat an air fryer basket with avocado oil and heat up air fryer to 400°F. Crack and beat eggs into a bowl and let sit. Add the spices, flax seed and almond flour into a second bowl and whisk until well mixed. Immerse each onion ring into the bowl with the egg wash until wholly coated.

2. Shake off excess and dip into the almond flour mixture until wholly covered. Transfer coated onion rings into a platter. Work in batches, add onion rings into the air fryer basket in one layer and coat lightly with avocado oil.

3. Cook for 5-7 minutes, turn and cook for 5 more minutes. Check every now and then to prevent burning. Repeat process with the remaining batches. Serve onion rings at once and enjoy.

Nutritional Information/Serving

Calories 77 kcal, Protein 3g, Carbs 4g, Fat 4g

Scrumptious Chocolate Brownies

Preparation Time: 10 minutes

Cook Time: 35 minutes

Serves: 6 servings

Ingredients

1/2 cup butter

1/2 cup chocolate chips, no-sugar added

1/4 cup erythritol

3 eggs

1 teaspoon vanilla extract

Method

1. Add chocolate and butter into an oven secure bowl and melt in a microwave for a minute. Note: do not overcook the chocolate. Stir the melted mixture thoroughly until combined.

2. Add vanilla, erythritol and eggs into a bowl and beat until frothy and light. Gradually add the chocolate mixture into the egg bowl and beat until mixture is combined and fully incorporated.

3. Pour batter into a prepared cake pan until an inserted toothpick comes out clean, for 20-30 minutes. Serve and enjoy.

Nutritional Information/Serving

Calories 224 kcal, Protein 4g, Dietary Fiber 1g, Carbs 3g, Fat 23g

Rich Air Fried Donuts

Preparation Time: 15 minutes

Cook Time: 10 minutes

Serves: 10 servings

Ingredients (donut)

1/4 cup heavy whipping cream

1/2 cup sour cream

1 teaspoon vanilla extract

4 big eggs

1/4 teaspoon nutmeg

1/2 cup coconut flour

1/4 cup erythritol

1/4 teaspoon baking soda

1 pinch salt

¼ cup avocado oil

Donut Coating

1 teaspoon cinnamon

1/4 cup erythritol

Method

1. Heat up air fryer to 355°. Add vanilla extract, eggs, whipping cream and sour cream into a big bowl and beat to combine. Gradually add the dry ingredients into the vanilla extract mixture and mix until well combined.

2. Pour batter into a donut pan, about 3/4 of the pan filled. Transfer donut pan into the fryer basket and cook until well cooked, for about 10-15 minutes. Move donuts from air fryer and let sit until cooled.

3. Add avocado oil into a skillet over med-heat. Add donuts into the hot oil and cook until golden brown, for about 2 minutes per side. Sprinkle cinnamon over donuts and serve.

Nutritional Information/Serving

Calories 141 kcal, Protein 4g, Total Carbs 2g, Total Fat 12g

Delicious Crispy Fried Pickles

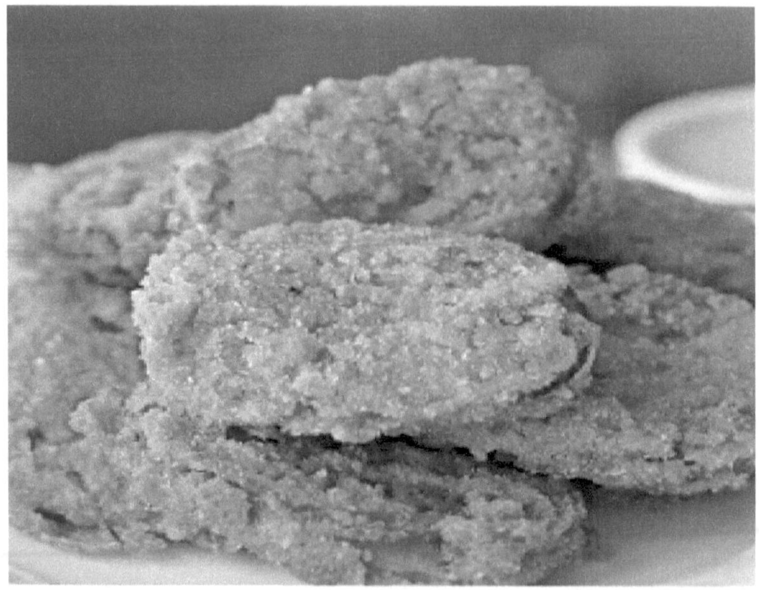

Preparation Time: 15 minutes

Cook Time: 6 minutes

Serves: 4 servings

Ingredients

3 tbsps (grated) parmesan cheese

1/2 cup pork rinds, crushed

1/2 cup almond flour

16 dill pickles, sliced

1 tsp avocado oil

1 (beaten) egg, large

Method

1. Add parmesan cheese and pork rind crumbs into a bowl and mix until combined. Add the beaten egg into another bowl. Add almond flour into a third bowl.

2. Immerse the pickle in the bow, with flour, move into the bowl with egg wash and lastly, dip into the crumb bowl. Coat the wire basket of an air fryer evenly. Add the breaded pickles into the air fryer basket in one layer.

3. Spray avocado oil over breaded pickles and cook at 370°F for 6 minutes. Remove, let sit to cool, serve and dig in.

Nutritional Information/Serving

Calories 155 kcal, Protein 17g, Fat 11g, Net Carbs 2g, Fiber 2g

Kale Chips

Preparation Time: 10 minutes

Cook Time: 7 minutes

Serves: 2 servings

Ingredients

2 tbsps avocado oil

1 bunch (get rid of hard spines and rip leaves into small pieces) kale, large

1/2 tsp salt

1/2 tsp chili powder

1/2 tsp pepper

Method

1. Add kale pieces into the wire basket of air fryer and coat with avocado oil and shake until wholly coated. Sprinkle pepper, salt and chili powder over

kale to season. Cook until desired doneness is reached, for 6-7 minutes at 360°F.

Nutritional Information/Serving

Calories 189 kcal, Protein 4.5g, Net Carbs 11.1g, Fat 14.4g

Crunchy Spinach Chips

Preparation Time: 5 minutes

Cook Time: 5 minutes

Serves: 2 servings

Ingredients

1 teaspoon avocado oil

1 bunch (remove stem and slice into small pieces) spinach

1/2 teaspoon salt

1/2 teaspoon garlic powder

Method

1. Heat up air fryer to 370°F. Add every ingredient into an average bowl and mix until combined. Add the seasoned spinach into the basket of the preheated air fryer. Cook spinach for 3 minutes. Shake and cook for 2 more minutes. Serve and enjoy.

Nutritional Information/Serving

Calories 37 kcal, Fat 1g, Protein 3g, Carbs 6g

Yummy Lemon Donuts

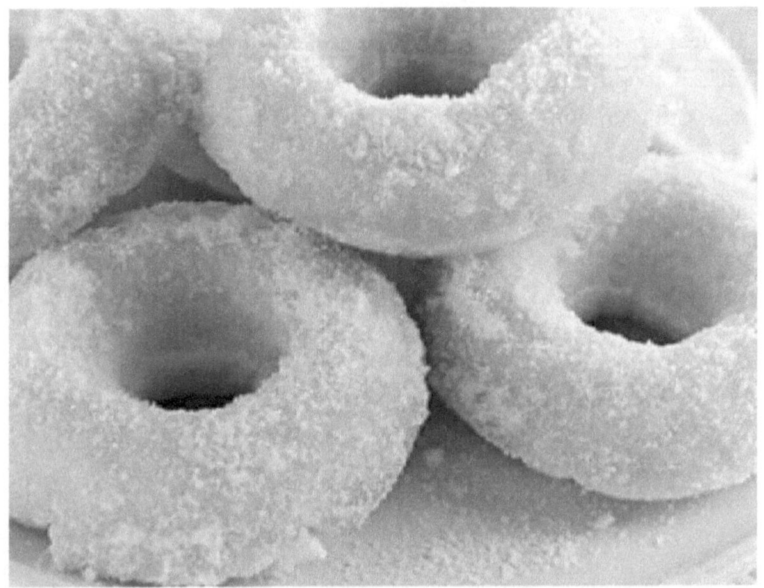

Preparation Time: 10 minutes

Cook Time: 10 minutes

Serves: 8 servings

Ingredients

4 tablespoons melted coconut oil

4 large eggs

2/3 cup lemon juice

3 tablespoons liquid stevia

1 teaspoon cinnamon

1 cup coconut flour

1 pinch salt

1 teaspoon baking soda

Method

1. Heat up air fryer to 350° and grease a donut pan with avocado oil. Add melted coconut oil, lemon juice, stevia, salt and eggs into a small bowl and whisk to combine. Add coconut flour, baking soda and cinnamon into a second bowl and sift to combine.

2. Add flour mixture into the lemon juice mixture until fully combined and a batter like consistency is reached. Pour batter into the prepared pan and spread equally. Place pan in the prepared fryer and cook for 10 minutes until donut edges become golden, at 350°.

3. Let sit to cool for 5-10 minutes before moving to a wire rack. Dribble with desired keto glaze.

Nutritional Information/Serving

Calories 179 kcal, Protein 5g, Dietary Fiber 0.2g, Carbs 9g, Total Fat 11.2

Crisped Zucchini Fritters

Preparation Time: 5 minutes

Cook Time: 30 minutes

Serves: 8 (2 fritter) servings

Ingredients (fritters)

2 tablespoon (divided) avocado oil

3 cups (squeeze out moisture) packed grated zucchini

6 tablespoons minced cilantro

2/3 cup diced onion

1 cup almond flour

3/4-1 teaspoon sea salt

1 egg white

Freshly ground black pepper

2 teaspoons coconut flour

Avocado oil

Lime Mayo Sauce

5 teaspoons fresh lime juice

1/2 cup mayo

Sea Salt, as necessary

4 teaspoons fresh chopped dill, tightly packed

Freshly ground black pepper

Method

1. Add squeezed zucchini into a big bowl. Add 2 teaspoons avocado oil into a big pan over med-heat. Add onions into the hot oil and cook until golden brown and tender. Add zucchini to the cooked onions.

2. Add coconut flour, almond flour, salt, cilantro and ground black pepper into the pan and stir to combine. Add egg white into the zucchini mixture and combine until zucchini is wholly coated. Heat up air fryer to 400°.

3. Spray fryer basket with avocado oil. Scoop several handfuls of the zucchini mixture. Working in batches, add about 4-5 zucchini fritter balls into the air fryer basket per time and spray top with avocado oil.

4. Cook fritters for about 10-15 minutes, until top is crisped and edges are golden brown. Flip fritters with a spatula and air fry for 5-7 more minutes.

Nutritional Information/Serving

Calories 222 kcal, Protein 3.8g, Dietary Fiber 2.8g, Total Carbs 6.9g, Total fat 21.8g

Nut Butter Glazed Donuts

Preparation Time: 10 minutes

Cook Time: 11 minutes

Serves: 6 servings

Ingredients

1/3 cup stevia powder

1 1/4 cups almond flour

1/2 tsp baking soda

1/2 tsp baking powder

1 egg

3/4 tsp salt

1 tsp vanilla

1/2 cup buttermilk

2 tbsps (melted and cooled) unsalted butter + 1 tbsp extra for topping

Glaze

2 tbsps milk

1/2 cup powdered stevia

1 pinch salt

2 tbsps peanut butter

Filling

1/2 cup blueberry jelly

Method

1. Add salt, baking soda, baking powder, stevia powder and almond flour into a big bowl and whisk until combined. Add vanilla, baking soda, baking powder and egg into another bowl and beat to combine.

2. Make a hole in the middle of the flour mixture and add the vanilla mixture. Mix mixture thorough until well combined. Add flour onto a counter top to prevent dough from sticking.

3. Knead and pat dough until a 3/4in thickness is reached on the prepared counter top. Cut out 3 1/2in rounds of dough from the flattened dough and coat with cooled butter. Cut a parchment paper round and place in a fryer basket.

4. Add dough into the prepared fryer basket and cook for 11 minutes at 350°. Add blueberry jelly into a squeeze bottle. Fill donuts with blueberry as desired. Add every glaze ingredient into a bowl, whisk to combine and dribble over donuts until coated.

Nutritional Information/Serving

Calories 250 kcal, Carbs 11g, Fat 21g, Protein 8g

Crispy Cheese Sticks

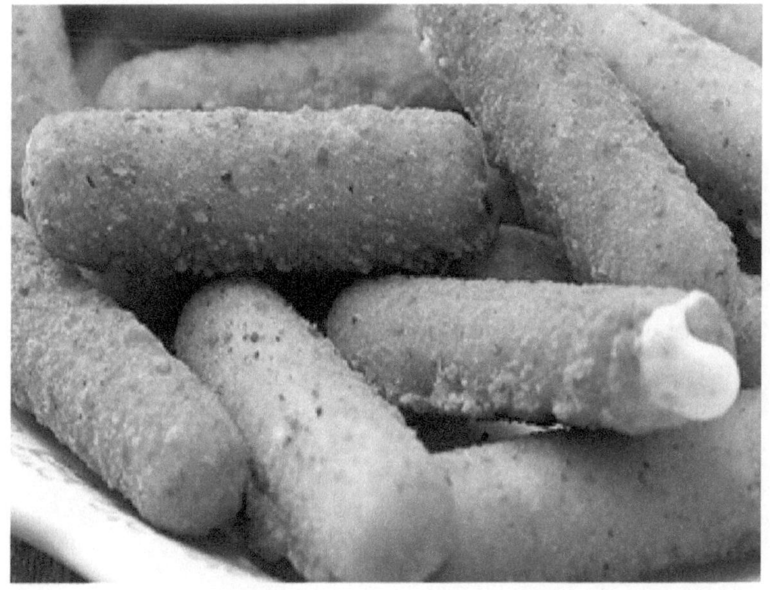

Preparation Time: 10 minutes

Cook Time: 10 minutes

Serves: 6 servings

Ingredients

2 (beaten) eggs, large

12 (string and cut in half) Mozzarella sticks

1/2 cup (powdered) parmesan cheese

1/2 cup almond flour

1/2 tsp garlic salt

1 tsp Italian seasoning

Method

1. Add garlic salt, Italian seasoning, parmesan cheese powder and almond flour into a bowl and mix until combined. Add eggs not a second bowl and whisk until combined. Coat each half of your cheese stick in the egg wash and transfer into the almond flour mixture until wholly coated.

2. Transfer breaded cheese stick into a well lidded container. Repeat process until every cheese stick is coated. Place the breaded cheese stick in the resealable container in a single layer. Place a parchment paper sheet over layer and top with another layer of cheese sticks.

3. Place well lidded cheese container into a freezer to chill for 30 minutes. Transfer chilled cheese sticks into the wire basket of an air fryer. Cook for 5 minutes at 400°F. After cooking, open air fryer basket and let cheese sticks sit for a minute.

4. Transfer cheese sticks to a platter before serving.

Nutritional Information/Serving

Calories 276 kcal, Fat 20g, Protein 18g, Carbs 4g

Limey Filled Artichokes

Preparation Time: 10 minutes

Cook Time: 30 minutes

Serves: 4 servings

Ingredients

1 tbsp avocado oil

1 (large) artichoke, cut stem off and trim a small part off the top

½ cup (crumbled) pork rinds

2 tbsps lime juice

¼ cup parmesan cheese, grated

½ cup (divided) mozzarella cheese, shredded

1 tsp minced garlic

2 tbsps fresh chopped cilantro

Salt and pepper, as necessary

Method

1. Add 1" of water into the base of a saucepan over med-heat, and bring to boiling. Add 2 tablespoons lime juice into the boiling water. Cut off the pointy and sharp end of the artichoke leaves using a kitchen scissors.

2. Transfer the artichokes into the boiling water, facing up. Place lid over saucepan and simmer until softened, for 25 minutes. Take artichoke out of the water, drain and let sit to cool.

3. Set aside few tbsps mozzarella cheese for later use. In the meantime, add chopped cilantro, crumbled pork rind, garlic, avocado oil, parmesan cheese and mozzarella cheese. Season with pepper and salt as necessary and stir until combined.

4. Scoop cheese mixture and stuff into the artichokes until filled. Scatter the reserved mozzarella cheese over artichoke. Heat up air fryer to 360°F. Sprinkle avocado oil over stuffed artichokes.

5. Place the stuffed artichokes in the wire basket of an air fryer and cook until desired doneness is reached, for 20 minutes.

Nutritional Information/Serving

Calories 137 kcal, Fat 9g, Protein 8g, Carbs 4g

SIDE DISHES

Delicious Radish Chips

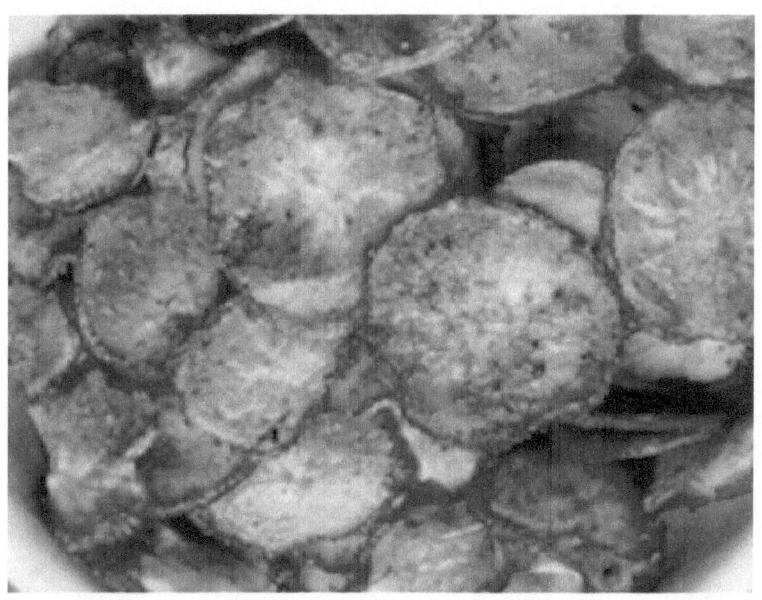

Preparation Time: 5 minutes

Cook Time: 20 minutes

Serves: 3 servings

Ingredients

1/2 teaspoon avocado oil

8-10 (wash, slice and pat dry) radishes

1/2 tsp onion powder and garlic powder

Salt and peppers, to taste

Method

1. Add radish slices to the wire basket of an air fryer in one layer and coat evenly with avocado oil. Sprinkle with onion powder, garlic powder, pepper, and salt. Seal air fryer.

2. Cook for 15-18 minutes at 390°F. Check radish chips at 7 minutes, shake air fryer basket and cook until desired doneness/crispness is reached.

Nutritional Information/Serving

Calories 35 kcal, Protein 1g, Net Carbs 2g, Fat 3g

Coconut Okra

Preparation Time: 15 minutes

Cook Time: 15 minutes

Serves: 4 servings

Ingredients

1 egg

8 oz. (remove stems and cut into 1/2" slices) fresh okra

1 cup pork rind crumbs

1 cup coconut milk

Avocado oil

1/2 tsp sea salt

Method

1. Add coconut milk and egg into an average bowl and beat until combined. Add okra slices into the milk mixture and stir until coated. Add salt and pork rind crumbs into a well lidded bowl and mix until combined.

2. Shake off excess milk mixture from the okra slices and add into the pork rind bowl. Shake until okra is wholly coated. Add okra slices into the wire basket of an air fryer and coat with avocado oil.

3. Cook for 5 minutes at 390°F. Shake air fryer basket and coat with oil again. Cook for 5 more minutes, shake air fryer basket and coat with avocado oil. Cook until okra slices are crisped and golden brown, for 2-5 more minutes.

Nutritional Information/Serving

Calories 188 kcal, Protein 11.9g, Total Carbs 2.3g, Fat 15g

Air Fried Asparagus

Preparation Time: 3 minutes

Cook Time: 7 minutes

Serves: 2 servings

Ingredients

1/4 teaspoon avocado oil

1 pound (cut off dry parts) asparagus

Salt and pepper, to taste

Method

1. Brush asparagus lightly with avocado oil and season with pepper and salt. Transfer the seasoned asparagus into the wire basket of an air fryer and cook at 400°F for 7 minutes. Shake air fryer basket midway during cooking.

2. Serve and enjoy.

Nutritional Information/Serving

Calories 46 kcal, Dietary Fiber 4.8g, Protein 5g, Net Carbs 4.1g, Fat 0.8g

Crisped Zucchini Gratin

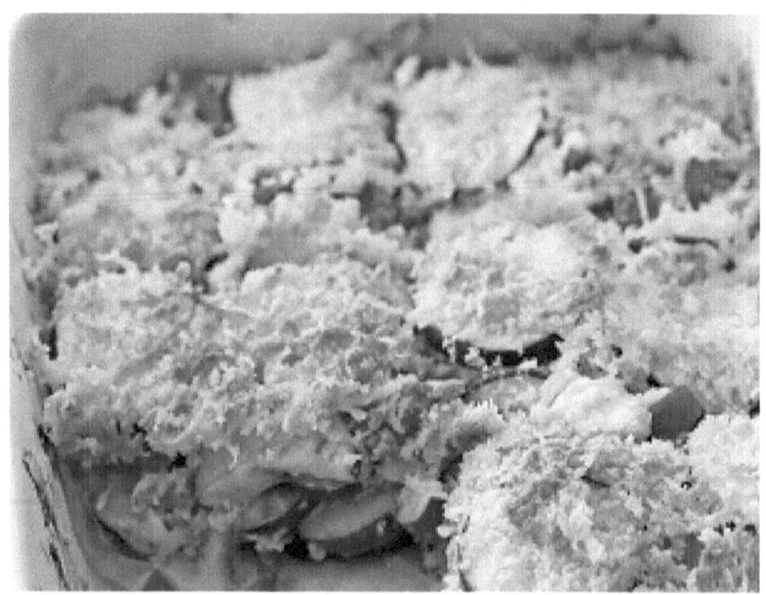

Preparation Time: 10 minutes

Cook Time: 15 minutes

Serves: 4 servings

Ingredients

1 tbsp fresh chopped cilantro

2 (halved lengthways and cut each half in two) zucchinis

4 tbsps pecorino romano cheese, grated

2 tbsps crumbled pork rinds

Salt and pepper, to taste

1 tbsp avocado oil

Method

1. Heat up air fryer to 350°F. Working in batches, add zucchini pieces into the wire basket of the air fryer. Add black pepper, avocado oil, pecorino romano cheese, pork rind and cilantro into a bowl and mix until combined.

2. Sprinkle half of cilantro mixture over first batch of zucchini and cook until golden brown, for 15 minutes. Repeat process with the remaining batch of zucchini and the remaining cilantro mixture. Serve and enjoy.

Nutritional Information/Serving

Calories 75 kcal, Protein 3.8g, Carbs 2.6g, Fat 5.6g

Roasted Onions & Sweet Peppers

Preparation Time: 15 minutes

Cook Time: 10 minutes

Serves: 4 servings

Ingredients

1 cup red bell pepper, sliced

1 cup green bell pepper, sliced

1 tbsp avocado oil

1 cup red onion, sliced

2 tbsps fresh chopped parsley

1/2 tsp salt

1 tbsp fresh lemon juice

Method

1. Heat up air fryer to 350°F. Add salt, avocado oil, onion and peppers into a big bowl and toss until wholly coated. Pour mixture into the wire basket

of an air fryer. Cook for 7-9 minutes, until onions are peppers are soft. Stir midway while cooking.

2. Pour air fried mixture into a serving bowl, add in lemon juice and parsley and toss until wholly coated. Serve and dig in.

Nutritional Information/Serving

Calories 55 kcal, Protein 0.8g, Carbs 5.6g, Fat 3.5g

Roasted and Crisped Brussels Sprouts

Preparation Time: 10 minutes

Cook Time: 20 minutes

Serves: 4 servings

Ingredients

1 tablespoon avocado oil

2 cups (halved and quartered into big chunks) brussels sprouts

1/4 teaspoon sea salt

Method

1. For 5 minutes, heat up air fryer to 375°F. Add sprout pieces into a big bowl and top with avocado oil. Toss mixture until wholly coated, transfer into the wire basket of the air fryer, and lightly coat basket with extra avocado oil.

2. Cook until desired crispiness is reached, for 9 minutes. Sprinkle with salt and let sit to cool. Repeat process with the remaining batch of sprouts.

Nutritional Information/Serving

Calories 50 kcal, Protein 1g, Fiber 2g, Net Carbs 2g, Fat 4g

Asparagus Spears with Mayo Sauce

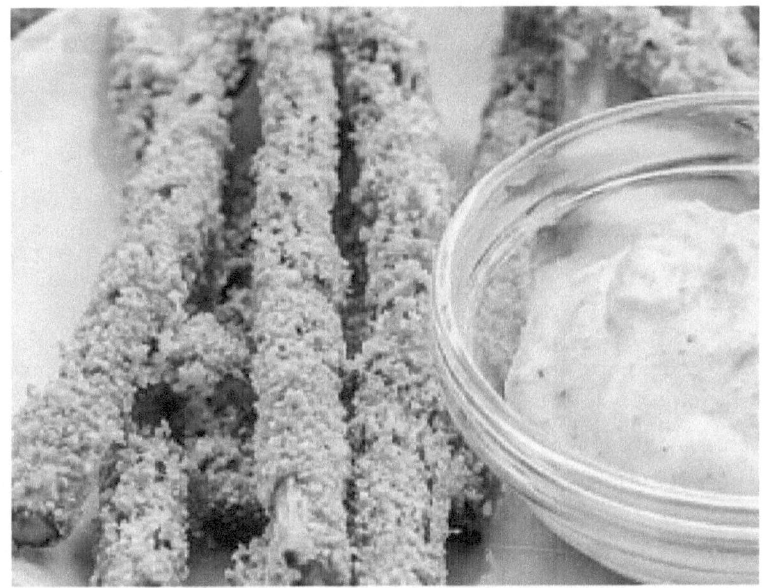

Preparation Time: 20 minutes

Cook Time: 5 minutes

Serves: 2 servings

Ingredients

Avocado oil

10 (trim off tough woody ends, rinse and pat dry) asparagus spears

1 tbsp heavy whipping cream

1 egg, large

1/3 cup pecorino romano cheese, finely grated

1/3 cup almond flour, blanched

1/2 tsp paprika

1/2 tsp salt

Sauce

1 tsp Dijon mustard

1/4 cup mayo

1/4 tsp black pepper

1/4 tsp cayenne

Method

1. Add cayenne, black pepper, mayo and Dijon mustard into a small bowl, stir until combined and place in a refrigerator until needed. Add heavy cream and egg into a bow and beat until combined. Transfer egg wash into a flat-bottomed bowl.

2. Add 1/2 tsp salt, 1/2 tsp paprika, 1/3 cup almond flour, and 1/3 cup pecorino romano cheese into a separate flat-bottomed bowl and stir until combined. Dip asparagus spears into the egg wash bowl until coated. Immerse asparagus spears into the almond flour mixture until wholly coated.

3. Transfer breaded asparagus onto a parchment paper lined plate and repeat process until no asparagus remains. Work in batches, transfer breaded asparagus spears into the wire basket of an air fryer. Spray avocado oil over spears and cook for about 5 minutes at 350°F.

4. Let sit to cool slightly. Serve at once with mayo sauce.

Nutritional Information/Serving

Calories 420 kcal, Protein 9g, Carbs 7g, Fat 40g

Roasted Cauliflower

Preparation Time: 10 minutes

Cook Time: 15 minutes

Serves: 2 servings

Ingredients

1 tbsp avocado oil

3 (halved and smashed) garlic cloves

1/2 tsp paprika, smoked

1/2 tsp salt

4 cups cauliflower florets

Method

1. Heat up air fryer to 400°F. Add paprika, salt, garlic and avocado oil into a bowl and combine. Add the cauliflower florets into the mixture and toss until wholly coated.

2. Transfer the coated cauli-florets into an air fryer basket and cook for 15 minutes, until crisp. Shake air fryer basket once every 5 minutes.

Nutritional Information/Serving

Calories 118 kcal, Protein 4.3g, Carbs 12.4g, Fat 7g

Air Fried Brussels Sprouts with Herbs

Preparation Time: 10 minutes

Cook Time: 8 minutes

Serves: 4 servings

Ingredients

1/2 teaspoons oregano, dried

1 pound (clean and trimmed) brussels sprouts

1 teaspoon garlic powder

1 teaspoon cilantro, dried

2 teaspoon avocado oil

1/4 teaspoon salt

Method

1. Add every ingredient into a big bowl and toss until sprouts is wholly coated. Add mixture into an air fryer basket and seal the lid. Cook for 8 minutes at 390°F. Let sit to cool before serving.

Nutritional Information/Serving

Calories 79 kcal, Protein 4g, Carbs 12g, Fat 2g

Lemon Roasted Broccoli with Pistachios

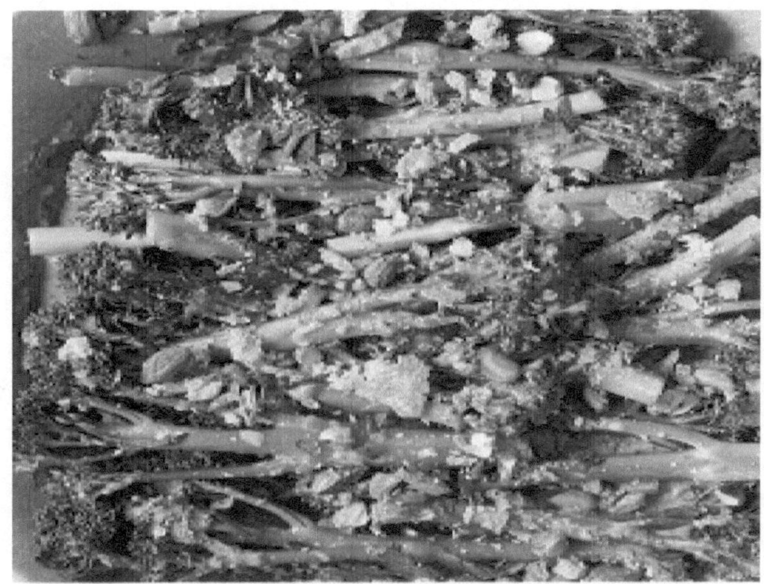

Preparation Time: 10 minutes

Cook Time: 20 minutes

Serves: 4 servings

Ingredients

1 1/2 tablespoon avocado oil

1 pound (cut into florets) broccoli

Salt

1 tablespoon minced garlic

2 teaspoons liquid stevia

2 tablespoons soy sauce, reduced sodium

1 teaspoon rice vinegar

2 teaspoons Sriracha

2 tbsp lemon juice

1/3 cup roasted salted pistachios

Method

1. Add broccoli florets, salt, garlic, and avocado oil into a big bowl and toss until whisky coated. Add broccoli into an air fryer basket in one layer, and cook for 15-20 minutes, until crisped and golden brown, at 400°F. Stir midway through cooking.

2. In the meantime, add rice vinegar, sriracha, soy sauce and stevia into a small heat-proof bowl and microwave until combined, for 10-15 seconds. Add the cooked broccoli into a bowl and top with the stevia mixture. Toss broccoli mixture until wholly coated.

3. Check for seasoning and adjust salt as necessary. Top with lemon juice and roasted pistachios.

Nutritional Information/Serving

Calories 156 kcal, Protein 4.3g, Carbs 6.2g, Fat 10.5g

Fried Broccoli with Herbs

Preparation Time: 10 minutes

Cook Time: 8 minutes

Serves: 4 servings

Ingredients

1/2 teaspoon sage, dried

1 pound (clean & trim) broccoli

1 teaspoon garlic powder

1 teaspoon cilantro, dried

2 tbsp avocado oil

1/4 teaspoon salt

Method

1. Add every ingredient into a big bowl and toss until broccoli is wholly coated. Pour mixture into the air fryer basket and seal the lid. Cook for 8 minutes at 400°F. Let sit to cool slightly before serving.

Nutritional Information/Serving

Calories 102 kcal, Protein 3.4g, Carbs 8.4g, Fat 7.1g

Air Fryer Haricot Verts

Preparation Time: 15 minutes

Cook Time: 10 minutes

Serves: 4 servings

Ingredients

3 (diced) bacon slices

3 cups (cut) haricot verts, frozen

1 tsp salt

1/4 cup water

1 tsp ground black pepper

Method

1. Add water, bacon pieces, frozen haricot verts into heat-safe pan and move pan into the wire basket of an air fryer. Cook for 15 minutes for 375°F> Adjust the temperature of the air fryer from 375°F to 400°F and cook mixture for 5 more minutes.

2. Sprinkle pepper and salt haricot verts mixture, and toss until combined. Take pan out of the air fryer basket, let sit and cover with a lid. Serve as desired and dig in.

Nutritional Information/Serving

Calories 95 kcal, Dietary Fiber 2g, Fat 6g, Protein 3g, Net Carbs 4g

END

Thank you for reading my book.

John Purcell

www.ingramcontent.com/pod-product-compliance
Lightning Source LLC
Chambersburg PA
CBHW031123250726
48655CB00004B/1820